SUFFERING PRESENCE

Suffering Presence

*Theological Reflections on Medicine,
the Mentally Handicapped,
and the Church*

STANLEY HAUERWAS

UNIVERSITY OF NOTRE DAME PRESS
NOTRE DAME, INDIANA 46556

Library of Congress Cataloging-in-Publication Data

Hauerwas, Stanley, 1940-
   Suffering presence.

   Includes bibliographies and index.
   1. Medical ethics.   2. Medicine—Religious aspects.
3. Mentally handicapped—Care and treatment—Moral and
ethical aspects.   I. Title.   [DNLM: 1. Ethics, Medical.
2. Mental Retardation.   3. Religion and Medicine.
W 50 H368s]
R725.5.H38   1986   174'.2   85-40603
ISBN 0-268-01721-2
ISBN 0-268-01722-0 (pbk.)

Contents

Preface

I hope this book exhibits my conviction that for whatever else ethics may be, moral reflection is barren unless it draws its substance from significant examples. That such a conviction is not widely shared today is at least in part due to the feeling that we lack significant examples. Yet I would contend such examples are all around us in the extraordinary lives of ordinary people who do what they have to do — such as caring for mentally handicapped people. Some years ago I was given the opportunity to have a small place in the world of the mentally handicapped by serving on the Board of the Council for the Retarded of St. Joseph County, Indiana. This book is but an attempt to develop systematically what those people — parents, workers, mentally handicapped alike — taught me. I, therefore, gratefully dedicate the book to them.

This is also a book about medicine, or better, about the care and courage I have seen exhibited by physician and patient in their joint effort to respond to illness. The recent development of "medical ethics" has had a certain crassness to it but it has nonetheless offered an opportunity for some of us to be part of the complex world of the sick and those who would care for them. I am indebted, therefore, to the many patients, nurses, physicians, and health care workers who have been willing to share their experiences with me. I owe a particular debt to the late Dr. Andre Hellegers for giving me my first opportunity to learn about the world of health and sickness. The footnotes in this book testify to how much I owe my philosophical and theological colleagues who have dedicated their lives to understanding this significant area of our experience.

I am aware that many will wonder why the world needs yet another collection of essays from me. Moreover, I admit to being a bit nervous about publishing too much, as I fear that the sheer bulk will become reason to ignore what I am about. My only defense is to say that I have brought these essays together because I think they develop a point

of view that has been largely absent in the vast literature on medicine
and medical ethics. It is true perhaps that I should take more time
to write books that are more coherent and to develop my argument
more carefully. But I have never pretended to be a "significant" thinker.
Rather I care about helping to sustain a conversation that will aid us
all in understanding the moral challenges that face us and how we
are to live best. I hope this book will be received in that spirit.

The many people who have made this book possible are literally
too numerous to mention. A few, however, must be named. Dr. Bonita
Raine, with whom one of these essays was co-authored, as the social
worker for the Protective Service Board of St. Joseph County taught
me how to be with the profoundly retarded. I remained her student
while I served as her dissertation director as she developed the
theological presuppositions necessary to sustain care of the retarded.
That Tom and Bernadette Merluzzi struggled to make the world more
hospitable for their daughter even as they fought with courage the
cancer that was to kill Bernadette will forever stay with me.

As usual I am in Jim Langford's debt for his willingness to welcome
my work for publication. He has taught me everything I know about
publishing and I am indeed fortunate to have such a teacher who is
also my friend. Mr. Greg Jones read and reread these essays making
many valuable suggestions for revision. Dr. Terry Tilley also read the
manuscript critically. The book would have no doubt benefitted even
more had I been able to do all he suggested. The book, however, is
better because Dr. Harmon Smith proposed a more intelligent way to
arrange the essays. For that and much else I am in his debt. My greatest
debt, however, is to Ann Rice, my editor at the University of Notre
Dame Press. I assure the reader that not only the writing but the substance of this book is better due to her annoying habit of finding the
weaknesses in my style as well as my argument. She made me work
more than I wanted, but I am in her debt for that.

As always I owe Anne and Adam everything, for they literally
make my life possible. They suffer my presence day in and day out,
not, I might add, without being a bit impatient with my considerable
shortcomings but also always with love. With their presence I am gifted
beyond measure.

Acknowledgments

The author and publisher are grateful to the following for permission to reprint:

Ethics in Science and Medicine for "Reflections on Suffering, Death, and Medicine," reprinted from vol. 6 (1979):229–237. © Pergamon Press Ltd 1979.

D. Reidel publishers of *Responsibility in Health Care*, ed. G. Asich, © 1982, for "Authority in Medicine."

D. Reidel publishers of *Theology and Medicine*, ed. Earl Shelp, 1985, for "Salvation and Health: Why Medicine Needs the Church."

New York Academy of Sciences for "Religious Concepts of Brain Death," reprinted from vol. 215 (1978): 329–338.

Alan Liss publishers of *Rights and Responsibilities in Modern Medicine*, ed. M. Basson, © 1981, for "Rational Suicide and Reasons for Living."

Linacre Quarterly for "Ethical Issues in the Use of Human Subjects," reprinted from the August 1975 issue.

Michael Glazier publishers of *The Deprived, the Disabled and the Fullness of Life*, ed. Flavian Dougherty, © 1984, for "Suffering the Retarded: Should We Prevent Retardation?"

The Furrow for "The Moral Challenge of the Handicapped," reprinted from the May 1981 issue, pp. 275–281.

Charles C. Thomas publishers of *Responsibility for Devalued Persons*, ed. S. Hauerwas, for "The Retarded, Society, and the Family: The Dilemma of Care," © 1982.

National Apostolate of the Mentally Retarded for "Community and Diversity: The Tyranny of Normality," reprinted from the Spring/Summer 1977 issue.

Introduction

The Rise (and Fall) of Medical Ethics

It is no secret that medical ethics has been the growth area in philosophical and theological ethics over the past two decades. There seems to be no end to conferences and books about ethics and medicine. Moreover, unlike most fads (intellectual and otherwise), enthusiasm and resources for the development of this new field have not abated. Like medicine itself, medical ethics seems to be self-generating. As long as people get sick they will need physicians, and it appears "bioethicists" are well on their way to convincing those who care for the sick that they need people around who are trained to think about the "ethics" of medicine.

How are we to account for this odd but, from the point of view of ethicists, welcome development? The most ready candidate to explain this phenomenon is the increasing technological power of modern medicine. We are now able to do what was once unimaginable and, it is often claimed, we are morally unprepared to respond. We may be able to keep an extremely premature child alive, but should we, since the very means to sustain life may also injure? Or should we encourage people to participate in experimental procedures in the hope of sustaining their lives for a short time by the use of mechanical hearts? These kinds of questions are occasioned by our technology, but as I hope to show in these essays the rise of "medical ethics" cannot be so simply explained. For our technological developments but reflect prior moral presuppositions about human life and how we should care for and preserve it.

In this book I argue that the rise of "medical ethics" is due more to the confused moral world we inhabit than to our technological revolution. "Medical ethics" therefore does not so much solve our difficulties as it reflects the moral anarchy of our times, for it is by no means clear how the practice of medicine can be sustained in a morally fragmented society. Put more strongly, it is by no means clear in such a society what the practice of medicine is about. Modern medicine's desperate attempt to cure through increasing use of technology may be but a way of avoiding the fact that it lacks any moral rationale for dealing with death's inevitability.

The upsurge of interest in medical ethics of course has been a godsend for ethicists. In a declining academic job market it has not only provided work for many ethicists — as now it seems every medical school needs to have its staff ethicist — but it also seems to have significant implications for how ethics is understood and done. For example, in his wonderfully titled article "How Medicine Saved the Life of Ethics," Stephen Toulmin argues that a concern with medicine has made it possible for philosophers to dispel the miasma of subjectivity surrounding contemporary ethical theory by forcing attention on objective and universal conditions all humans share — i.e., sickness, reproduction, death, etc.

Moreover, Toulmin contends the attention of medicine to specific cases has provided philosophers with the opportunity to rediscover the importance of casuistry. For it turns out that the problems of clinical medicine and applied ethics are but varieties of a common mode of reflection.

> In both fields, theoretical generalities are helpful to us only up to a point, and their actual application to particular cases demands, also, a human capacity to recognize the slight but significant features that mark off, say, a "case" of decent reticence from one of cowardly silence. Once brought to the bedside, so to say, applied ethics and clinical medicine use just the same Aristotelean kinds of practical reasoning, and a correct choice of therapeutic procedure in medicine is the *right* treatment to pursue, not just as a matter of medical technique but for ethical reasons also. ([2], p. 743)

Toulmin also notes that attention to medicine has challenged the radical individualism that has dominated so much of contemporary ethical reflection. That individualism combined with a stress on "rights" and free choice meant all role-dependent obligations could only appear as morally deficient. As a result the specific code of responsibilities any profession lays on its practitioners has at times seemed lost, or worse, denied. By attending to the professions, however, we can recover some of our lost sense of community for at the present time, our professional commitments have taken on many of the roles that our communal commitments used to play. Even people who find moral philosophy generally unintelligible usually acknowledge and respect the specific ethical demands associated with their own professions or jobs, and this offers us some kind of a foundation on which to begin reconstructing our view of ethics. For it reminds us that we are in no position to fashion lives for ourselves, purely as individuals. ([2], p. 745)

Finally, Toulmin suggests that the physician-patient relationship can help us recover the Aristotelean insight that there is a close connection between relationships and how we describe as well as understand actions. For within different relationships the very same deeds or words can represent quite different acts. "Words that would be a perfectly proper command from an officer to an enlisted man, or a straightforward order from a master to a servant, might be a humiliation if uttered by a father to a son, or an insult if exchanged between friends" ([2], p. 747). That such is the case means that ethics is forced to reconsider the significance of reasonableness as central to the moral life. For it is in medicine that we learn that general principles, by themselves, never settle ethical issues, but we can grasp the force of principles only as we see them applied to particular situations.

While I am sympathetic with Toulmin's argument, I think our actual situation is more ambiguous. I am sure he is right, in principle, to suggest that ethics has much to learn from medicine, but I am not convinced that in fact our way of reflecting about the moral life has been transformed by the recent turn toward medical ethics. Indeed, I think in many ways the signs point in the opposite direction, particularly as we consider theological ethics.

Medicine in many ways did save the life of ethics, but not by redirecting our methodological assumptions in the manner Toulmin suggests. For example, many of the books written in medical ethics look just like standard introductory texts in general ethics. They have the required chapters dealing with the autonomy of the individual and the conceptual condition necessary to insure the objectivity of ethical judgments. Then there are the chapters on normative theory which highlight the strengths and weaknesses of teleological and deontological theories of moral obligation. A chapter on patient-physician relations usually follows, and the dilemma of paternalism is gone over yet again.

All this is followed by the required chapters on death and dying, truth-telling, experimentation, and so on.

What is remarkable about such books is not that they are badly done. Indeed many of them are done very well. What is remarkable is that confrontation with medicine has had almost no effect on how philosophers and theologians continue to think about ethics. Rather than letting the substantive moral presuppositions and practices involved in medicine challenge their explanatory paradigm about morality, philosophers and theologians went on working just as they always had; they just changed their examples. Rather than testing deontological or utilitarian theories by considering what you do when you have a fat person caught in the entrance of a cave so that all left in the cave will die unless the fat person is blown up, they turn to examples of scarce medical resources. Contrary to Toulmin's contention, ethics has continued to be done pretty much the way it was prior to medicine becoming the object of ethical reflection.

Moreover, physicians have been fairly satisfied with this. Confronted by issues that seemed morally troubling, physicians began to acknowledge that medicine must again touch base with ethics. As a result many failed to notice that medicine was first and foremost a moral practice constituted by intrinsic moral convictions that are operative even if not explicitly acknowledged. As people who had been taught to think of themselves as experts and to trust other experts, they turned to experts in "ethics" to help them think about the moral challenges with which they seemed to be faced. It never occurred to them that the very idea of the "expert" might be problematic and even more so when applied to an area like ethics. But "ethicists" at least sounded like experts with their talk about metaethics and distinctions between teleological and deontological modes of justification. And so physicians went to school at the feet of contemporary ethical theory, believing that if they attended to such distinctions they might be helped to make more "rational" and "objective" moral decisions. As a result they failed to see that the very "ethics" they were learning might make them overlook, and perhaps even distort, the already substantive moral commitments that are constitutive of and embodied in their daily care of patients.

Toulmin suggests that attention to medicine has forced ethics to take seriously the significance of role-specific duties. I have no doubt that serious attention to the patient-physician relation *should* have that effect, but I think the exact opposite has taken place. Instead physicians have been urged by "ethicists" to understand their duties to their patients as but instances of more general and universal obligations that pertain between any persons. Construal of the physician-patient relation in these terms, moreover, has been heralded as a moral advance against physician paternalism. I have no interest in defending the often overbearing attitude of physicians toward their patients, but the proposed cure strikes me as almost worse than the illness itself. In particular when the relation between a physician and patient is construed as a contractual relation between autonomous individuals, the temptation to construe medical care in terms of capitalist notions of property becomes almost irresistable, corrupting physician and patient alike.

Therefore if medicine saved the life of ethics, it did so by breathing new life into what was becoming an increasingly questionable activity. Indeed the very assumption that "ethics" is a specifiable discipline was beginning to be questioned, as well as the assumption (accepted for far too long) that something called metaethics can really insure the objectivity of ethicists. Those very assumptions, however, gained new life as "ethics" rushed to show their relevance to the new challenge presented by medicine.

But if medicine was a "godsend" for philosophers, it was even more so for theologians who worked in ethics. If philosophers working in ethics were beginning to face some of the limits of their methodological presuppositions, theologians were having trouble discovering if they even *had* an identifiable method when it came to ethics. Medicine seemed to offer an opportunity to escape from the interminable ambiguity associated with being a theological thinker concerned about ethical matters. Issues in medicine could be addressed without having to worry about how religion might or might not relate to morality. "Religious ethicists" could turn to medicine using the same terms as the philosophers and be rewarded for how useful their analysis was, even though their theological presuppositions were not brought into play. Theological ethics when applied to medicine becomes but another example of "quandary ethics" on the assumption that ethics primarily involves clear thinking about hard cases.

All of this is but a long way to explain why I have brought these essays together in a book. I have done so not because I think the world needs another book in medical ethics. As these essays will make clear I am not even sure if I believe in "medical ethics" as a specifiable discipline or area. Moreover these essays do not pretend to treat the full range of matters involved for an adequate account of medicine as a moral practice. Rather I have brought them together because I think they do exemplify a point of view that is an alternative to much of the work currently being done in medical ethics. For I have made no attempt to hide my theological presuppositions, and instead have tried to show how those presuppositions can illuminate the care we offer one another through the office of medicine.

Many who turn their attention to medicine for moral analysis do so with reforming zeal. It is their intention to challenge the status of physicians and of the medical establishment in general. One of the worst things you can say about a "medical ethicist" is that he or she is soft on physicians. While I am sure that much needs changing about the current institutional form our medical practice takes, my first interest is not to reform but to understand what it is physicians and patients do when they make themselves available to one another in times of illness and crisis. If that makes me "soft" on physicians, so be it. However I have found that what physicians often say normally about the practice of medicine fails to do justice to the profound moral conviction already involved in the practice of medicine. In fact one of my aims is to try to help physicians and patients alike to make explicit what we are doing insofar as we participate in the common practice we call medicine.

As Toulmin suggests, I think medicine may be one of the most telling contexts for uncovering some of our most profound moral commitments as a community. In these essays I have tried in particular to suggest that fundamental to understanding the moral art of medicine is the willingness of patient and physician alike to be present to one another in times of suffering. (By *physician* I mean all called to be with and aid the sick. I realize *physician* may be associated too strictly with doctors but it seems preferable to "health-care providers.") We assume that a physician should be available to the ill. After all, that is his or her job. But we forget the profound moral presupposition that underlies that "job description," namely that illness does not quarantine a person from the human community. On the contrary, the community should be present to the ill even as they suffer. Such an observation may well strike many as so obvious it need not be said, but I hope that the present essays will at least help dispel the assumption that the obvious is any less morally significant because it is obvious.

Moreover, I believe that questions raised by medical care are precisely those that most require theological resources. As Tristram Engelhardt observes, quoting T. S. Eliot, " 'Birth and copulation, and death. That's all the facts when you come to brass tacks.' Since medicine touches on these three, and illness as well, the bioethical reflections they occasion will touch on our central human concerns" ([1], p. 76). It is not only medicine that touches on those "brass tacks," but religion does as well. That medicine and religion are interrelated cannot be avoided. The interesting project is understanding how. It is my hope that these essays make some contribution to that endeavor.

Medicine involves the needs and interests that we all share. All of us wish to avoid untimely death. All wish to avoid unnecessary suffering. All wish to be cared for when we are hurt. These basic interests or needs, as Toulmin suggests, do have a kind of almost inescapable "objectivity," making medicine an especially interesting testing ground for theological ethics. Medicine provides a powerful reminder to Christians of our "nature" as bodily beings beset by illness and destined for death. Yet medicine also reminds us it is our "nature" to be a community that refuses to let suffering alienate us from one another. The crucial question is what kind of community we should be to be capable of that task.

This is particularly important for the kind of ethic I have tried to develop in my work—that is, an ethic that is specifically Christian. Many have suggested that such an ethic is inherently sectarian in a world like ours, since a religious ethic can have no "universal" foundation or starting point. Yet, as I hope these essays make clear, the particularistic starting point from which I begin in no way prevents me from addressing issues in medicine and/or how medicine involves questions of public policy.

Thinking Theologically about Bioethics in a Pluralist Society

The question of the relation of medicine, public policy, and theology is extremely complex. From the perspective I develop here the question is not what should be our public policy concerning medicine, but rather how, in a pluralist society, we might sustain the public policy which medicine already embodies. Too often we forget that the mere fact a society makes it possible for some of its number to dedicate

their lives to care for the ill is already a significant public policy, though
it may well be one that is increasingly hard to sustain in a secular and
pluralist society.

For such an understanding of medicine assumes that medicine
is a practice with internal goods and standards of excellence that give
it a moral intelligibility unlike most of our institutions. In a sense
medicine represents a sectarian commitment about how to care for the
ill. Allen Verhey has reminded us that the Hippocratic Oath did not
originally reflect a broad consensus, but only the convictions of a small
group of Pythagorean physicians late in the fourth century B.C. As
Verhey points out, however,

> the oath's prohibitions of active euthanasia, of assisting in suicide, and
> of abortion were not argued on the basis of Pythagorean premise; they
> were given as standards of practice whose telos is to benefit the sick.
> Because the ends intrinsic to medicine are to heal the sick, to protect
> and nurture health, to maintain and restore physical well-being, limits
> could be imposed on the use of skills within the practice. The skills
> may not be used to serve alien ends, and the destruction of human
> life, either the last of it or the first of it, is an alien and conflicting
> end. The point was not that one would fail to be a good Pythagorean
> if one violated these standards, although that is true enough, but rather
> that one would fail to be a good medical practitioner. The good physi-
> cian is not a mere technician; he is committed by the practice of
> medicine to certain goods and to certain standards. ([3], p. 159)

It is not my purpose to argue that the practice of medicine so
understood can be sustained only in terms of Christian commitments.
The very fact that the Hippocratic Oath was developed from non-
Christian sources is enough to defeat any such claim. As Verhey argues,
however, given Christian convictions about the care of the weak as well
as the centrality of gratitude, it is not surprising that Christians found
the Hippocratic Oath useful to express their own commitments.[1] The
oath is a form of "natural" morality in which Christians rightly believe
they continue to have a stake. As I argue in essay 2, medicine so
understood embodies the wisdom of the body that is essential to the
moral as well as the physical health of our society.

Yet it is just this conception of medicine that the development
of bioethics seems to deny. No one has put the matter more clearly
than H. Tristram Engelhardt in his "Bioethics in Pluralist Societies."
Engelhardt notes that bioethics as a field must be understood as the

attempt to develop an ethic suitable to a secular society. Such an ethic must find the means to maintain a peaceable community where there are competing conceptions of the good, without recourse to totalitarian strategies. The fundamental project, then, is to frame "an understanding of how a society will deport itself in conditions when one view of the good life, or of the nature of man, will not be imposed by force on all." ([1], p. 65)[2]

Engelhardt suggests that the passage into such a community will be painful for many who believe in a religion or in the power of a particular culture. They must always live between two worlds: that of their particularistic convictions — what Engelhardt calls their "private conscience" — and the public morality necessary for maintaining a peaceable community. Such a stance is especially painful in terms of medical ethics, since medicine touches on those matters about which our "private conscience" cares so much.

Yet medicine has no choice in a pluralist culture to be anything other than a secular profession, he claims. In order to care for Christians, Jews, Muslims, and atheists alike, medicine has had to fashion or conform to a secular morality that accents respect for freedom. It does this by focusing more on procedures such as free and informed consent than on substantive moral convictions dealing with such matters as abortion or suicide. The latter must now be regarded as matters of private choice, not to be made by the profession or the community.

With admirable clarity Engelhardt draws out the implications of the development of such a secular morality and medicine. He quite rightly suggests that it necessarily requires the subordination of private morality to the general purposes of the public morality. Thus we should not be surprised that we are developing a public morality regarding such matters as sexuality, abortion, and dying that is in tension with the morality of our more particularistic religious communities.

> Commitment to the respect of freedom and recognition of a pluralism of views regarding the good life have their implications. These implications suggest that the custodians of the moral order of the next century will, should we live freely, be like good bureaucrats who follow procedures respecting the freedom of a nation's citizens without imposing a particular view of the good life. One might think here of a mail carrier who delivers with equal reliability the *New England Journal of Medicine*, *Playboy*, and the *Journal of Medicine and Philosophy*. ([1], p. 66)

Of course one of the primary "custodians" Engelhardt has in mind is medicine.

The procedural nature of the morality of secular society should not, however, be dismissed as lacking moral substance. For, as Engelhardt points out, such a morality affirms the centrality of respect for freedom in the moral life. Since freedom functions as the moral core of the logic of pluralism, we are bound to respect the free choices of individuals no matter what those choices may be. Only those who resist becoming "the agents of freedom" and reserve the right to use force to impose their views on others are to be prevented from doing what they wish. What all must recognize, if they are to avoid being outlaws in the peaceable community, is that any concrete view of the moral life turns on intuitions that are not shared by all. Therefore citizens in a society like ours must be committed to resolving disputes through the procedural means necessary to safeguard freedom.

To respect freedom as the core of the moral life means we will be compelled morally to tolerate the loss of some important moral goods, since there can be no way to embody in public policy any good that is contentious — e.g., you cannot force parents to secure life-saving surgery for their children. Moreover physicians may choose to provide services that many hold to be immoral. In Engelhardt's peaceable community, however, physicians' primary role will be that of mediators among individuals possessing varying perspectives on the good. The physician's task will be to provide "a map showing the likely consequences of various choices, without insisting where the person must go, what the patient must choose as his or her therapy style, sickness style, or death style" ([1], p. 70).

The emphasis on freedom, moreover, underwrites the modern view that we are most nearly "natural" when we are intervening to transcend the "natural" constraints on human behavior. Nothing embodies this ethic more fully than the change in sexual ethics occasioned by the development of contraception. In such an ethos medicine does not try to help us come to terms with the constraints of nature, but rather "enables free individuals to achieve the biological destinies they choose, as, for example, within the area of reproduction" ([1], p. 72). In doing so, however, a subtle shift has taken place: freedom is not only respected as a condition for a moral order but is seen as a value that makes us more nearly what we should be — namely, a biological species whose characteristic is to change over time.

The development of successful biomedical technology, therefore, is but the moral manifestation of this new ethos. But with this expanding power comes the expansion of responsibility. The birth of a child is no longer a gift of God but an event for which we can be held accountable. The same is true of sickness and death.

> Given the growing costs of prolonged high-technology care, we may come to consider the use of living wills, and the refusal of life-saving treatment which assures little quality of life, as morally exemplary. An ethos is likely to develop showing some likeness to Seneca's letter on suicide, enjoining us to take responsibility for the time and the circumstances of our death. This is but to underscore a general theme: increase of power over ourselves will increase our responsibility concerning ourselves. ([1], p. 75)

Engelhardt does not mean his arguments for a secular morality to replace religious and other more particularistic moralities. The latter, however, constitute the "soft dimension of ethics" by instructing us when and under what circumstances it would be good to reproduce, have an abortion, refuse life-saving treatment. But these particularistic understandings will need to be set within the context and protection of the secular morality. This may well force those who have convictions at odds with the "ethos of freedom" to live in two moral worlds: "that of particular communities and that of secular public morality. There will be an unavoidable moral schizophrenia. Truthfulness of heart will force us always to embrace more than one moral stance. One cannot choose one or the other. One must embrace both" (]1], pp. 76–77).

Yet if we embrace both, as Engelhardt admits, we will have transformed the character of our religious convictions. For now they are subordinate to the ethos of freedom that, Engelhardt rightly argues, cannot help but become a whole way of life. That such is the case helps us understand why the development of bioethics has had such ambiguous results for theological thinkers. Inasmuch as they wanted to address the issues raised by medicine in terms amenable to our liberal society, they have had to use the language and concepts of Engelhardt's peaceable community. Ironically, in attempting to show the relevance of religious convictions for bioethics by theologically underwriting the ethos of freedom, theologians have been digging their own grave and, as I hope these essays show, undermining the ethos necessary to make medicine an intelligible moral practice.

They have done so because there seemed to be no other alternative. As Engelhardt notes, to try to argue seriously from a theological perspective seems to put one in a totalitarian camp. Moreover, who could possibly be against contraception in an age of freedom? Engelhardt is quite right that all the cultural forces appear to be on the side of those who would have us increasingly intervene in "nature" in the interest of expanding our sphere of freedom. Theologically it seems to be a necessary survival strategy for religious thinkers to support the ethos of freedom. After all, most "religious people" in our society believe deeply in the ethos of freedom. A few may remain nervous that we must begin to encourage people to choose their death "style," since it would seem to require physicians to begin to help people die rather than live, but such nervousness is but a cultural lag in a community that has insufficiently embodied the ethos of freedom.

For me to insist on the significance of theological convictions for understanding and sustaining the practice of medicine, therefore, looks like a step in the wrong direction. It is a failure to live by the requirements of a peaceable community. At least as such a community is construed by Engelhardt, it is nothing less than a declaration of war. Of course Engelhardt is not suggesting we must give up our religious convictions, but only for matters of public policy we must consider those convictions secondary or private. Yet I cannot accept that compromise, since to do so would be to deny that such convictions have any interesting truth value. Moreover, as I suggested above, such a compromise would decisively change the moral character of medicine as a profession determined by an internal ethic.

Though these essays were written prior to Engelhardt's article, they presuppose and try to address the position he has developed so well. While I think Engelhardt's argument is normatively wrong, I have no doubt that his position is descriptively powerful. That is, I am sure that the ethics he describes as well as the corresponding form of medicine is coming into being. One of my primary aims in these essays is simply to suggest the implications of such an ethic, to see whether, in fact, we are willing to so live. I suspect most accept the ethos of freedom because they continue to rely on presuppositions of past particularistic moralities that are slowly being destroyed by Engelhardt's public morality. In other words, Engelhardt's mail-carrier-like physician is possible only because at heart we believe that physicians will continue to embody virtue correlative to the internal ethics of medicine. But if a physician is only a high-powered mail carrier, there is no rationale to support this belief.

I have therefore tried to give quite a different account of medicine than that presented by Engelhardt. Rather than being a group of highly trained technocrats waiting for their customers to determine what service they wish to have performed, I have tried to sketch the essential moral presuppositions necessary for sustaining the claim that medicine is a moral art and thus deserving of the designation "profession." The very willingness of the physician to be present in times of illness and the ill to avail themselves of the physician constitutes a morality that simply cannot be explained on Engelhardt's terms. Of course he can respond that such commitments are not essential for medicine, but at least we ought to be aware that if he is right, we have not only changed medicine but morally the kind of people and community we once thought we ought to be.

If any one intuition underlies these essays it is the recognition of what an extraordinary gesture it is for a society to set aside some to dedicate their lives to the care of the ill. That we do so, I think, is not primarily because we are self-interested and thus want to guarantee that when we are ill we will not be abandoned, but because we are unwilling to abandon others who need help. Therefore medicine as a moral practice draws its substance from the extraordinary moral commitment of a society to care for the ill. Medicine, as many of its critics like to point out, may have little significance for insuring the health of a population. (Effective sanitation is much more important for the health of a population than medicine.) But the care we provide to individuals through the office of medicine is no less morally significant for that. Even when medicine cannot cure, the care physicians provide is all the more important.

Contrary to being part of Engelhardt's ethos of freedom, therefore, I think medicine as a profession inherently carries the wisdom of our finitude. I don't mean to imply that I am opposed to all attempts to make us less subject to the limits of our nature. What I object to is the justification of those attempts solely in the name of freedom.[3] For such freedom too often turns out to be but a name for the power that some exercise unjustly against others—for example, the termination of pregnancies solely in the name of freedom to do what we want with "our" bodies. Rather than being about such freedom, medicine still carries what I call the wisdom of the body, through which we learn to negotiate the limits and possibilities of this existence in a just and caring fashion.

I have not tried to argue that such a view of medicine necessarily requires theological presuppositions in order to subsist. Indeed I do not believe it does. However I have suggested that such a medicine may well require a community to sustain its practice, particularly in a world such as the one depicted by Engelhardt. While not "sectarian" in my intent, I do think the kind of medicine I try to portray in these essays will become increasingly difficult in a society dedicated to freedom as the overriding value. Yet the medicine I have tried to describe I take to be that which accords best with the kind of people we are meant to be. If a medicine so constituted appears sectarian in Engelhardt's peaceable community, that says at least as much about the moral limits of his community as it does about my conception of medicine.

Yet Engelhardt can rightly ask how I intend to sustain, in a pluralistic society, a medicine formed by those substantive convictions which I have suggested are internal to it. Would it not in fact be dependent on his peaceable society in which my particularities, as well as others, are allowed to flourish? To reject his account of community seems to threaten anarchy and possibly even violence. I think that is not the case, however, as I believe a peaceable community is finally possible, not when there is merely a willingness to live and let live, but only when freedom is supported by a profound commitment to the protection and care of each person's life (i.e., a commitment to those very convictions I have suggested are intrinsic to the practice of medicine as a moral art).

This is not just another way of affirming Engelhardt's ethos of freedom in different language. In contrast to Engelhardt, I do not pretend that freedom is all we need. In my view freedom is possible and meaningful only when it is correlated with convictions about the kind of people we ought to be, as well as the kind of institutions we ought to support. Those in the practice of medicine ought to expect parents of mentally handicapped children to care for them. While this view may well appear coercive, it is no more so than Engelhardt's ethos of freedom. For when freedom and its enhancement becomes an end in itself, we lose any account of human life that gives content and direction to freedom. As a result we end by being less rather than more free.

Why the Mentally Handicapped?

But why the mentally handicapped? This is not just a book on medicine, for some of the essays deal with mental retardation with little reference to medicine. What does mental retardation have to do with the kind of issues I have discussed above? I think once anyone has read through these essays that relationship will be more evident. However, at least some response should be made at this point.

The most obvious answer is that the mentally handicapped are both helped by and suffer from medical care. Because of their handicap they are among those in our society who are at the mercy of the "health-care" system. They, therefore, become one way of focusing on many of the problems in medical ethics. More importantly, however, I have tried to show how medicine's dealing with them gives us indications about the moral presuppositions that in general shape medical practice. Issues such as our attitude to suffering, what we understand health to be, the place of the family in determining the care of children, the relation between caring and curing, quickly come to the surface when dealing with the mentally handicapped. In short, the mentally handicapped simply make and raise extremely interesting problems.

That they do so presents a dilemma, for I fear that my use of the retarded in these essays is but another example of the disrespect with which they are often treated. Am I merely "using" them to bolster my arguments? I cannot pretend to have avoided such a result, but I hope that at least some of these essays help us understand better what profound moral presuppositions are operative in a family which simply accepts the fact that they should care for their mentally handicapped child. Moreover, I hope I have been able to show that such a commitment is not unlike the kind needed for upholding the practice of medicine, for medicine reflects, as well as depends on, societal presuppositions to sustain its craft. It does not make *some* difference which community supports the practice of medicine, it makes *all* the difference.

Yet a community with substantive commitments is increasingly difficult to find in our society. Engelhardt's ethos of freedom gives no direction about how children born handicapped should be treated. Frequently they are regarded as "limits" that prevent the full flowering of a society dedicated to expanding our range of choices. The mentally handicapped cannot help but appear anomalous in a society formed by the ethos of freedom. But then so does a medicine committed to being present to the ill when there is little chance of cure. Therefore by focusing on the mentally handicapped I hope at the same time to have illuminated some of the moral challenges facing medicine in an ethos of freedom.

I should mention that I have used interchangeably "mentally handicapped" and "retarded." The former term is obviously preferable but it is also ambiguous. Many suppose that "mentally handicapped" suggests mental illness. Of course someone mentally retarded could also be mentally ill, but it would be a terrible mistake to underwrite the idea that mental retardation and mental illness are necessarily related.

I assume, however, one ought to use the language that those who are so labeled prefer. Thus in the title of the book I have used the phrase "mentally handicapped," because mentally handicapped people have made it clear to me that they prefer such a designation if we insist on labeling them. I should have gone over each essay to be consistent, but I did not because I think it important that the essays reflect something of the cultural limits in which such matters must be discussed. At one time people suffering from some kind of mental limit were called idiots or imbeciles, certainly pejorative designations. It was thought a more "scientific" term such as "retardation" was preferable and might avoid some of the self-fulfilling aspects of the more negative designation. But it seems no term can avoid the general negative response our culture places on those whose mental life does not correspond to what we assume is normal. I know of no way to avoid this problem but can only call our attention to it.

The Character of These Essays

The essays that comprise this book have been written over a number of years and for quite diverse occasions and audiences. I have made no attempt to disguise their character as such nor will I make any exaggerated claims for their interdependence. However I have tried to group them in the manner that best highlights my central thesis. Moreover, I have made revisions to promote their coherence.

The essays in "Medicine as a Moral Art" develop my argument that medicine is a profession determined by the moral commitment to care for the ill. I realize such a claim appears so obvious one can only wonder why anyone should think it interesting or important. However, as I try to show, the ability to sustain such care in the face of suffering and death is no easy enterprise, for the constant temptation is to try to eliminate suffering through the agency of medicine rather than let medicine be the way we care for each other in our suffering. Indeed I suspect the increasing technological character of medicine with the correlative growth of specialization reflects the attempt to substitute scientific expertise for the moral commitment necessary to maintain medicine as a coherent profession.

A word, perhaps, needs to be said about essay number 2. That essay is a bit denser than most in the book. However for my argument it is the crucial essay, because it considers why those who practice the craft of medicine are rightly regarded as having authority. To make that case I am forced to develop a constructive thesis about the nature of authority and why certain professions should have such authority granted to them. In fact this essay is as much an exercise in political theory and epistemology as it is about medicine. I think, however, that the position I try to develop in this chapter will make increasing sense in the light of the rest of the book. As I try to show in the succeeding chapter, the moral commitments that constitute medicine as a profession can be sustained only if a people exist who are convinced that the good intrinsic to medicine — what I call "the wisdom of finitude" — is but part of the good they hold in common.

The essays in the second section are similar insofar as they deal with the kind of concrete problems normally associated with medical ethics — i.e., definition of death, suicide, informed consent, proxy consent, and *in-vitro* fertilization. Yet that is not why I have grouped these essays together. For in each I have tried to show how attempts to deal with these issues in terms of the kind of medical ethics Engelhardt recommends have been insufficient because substantive convictions embodied in a distinct community's habits and institutions could not be presupposed. Thus we attempt to develop technical definitions for determining when someone is "really dead," because we lack any common sense of what a good death might look like. In like manner we have emphasized informed consent as the crucial issue for determining the legitimacy of experimentation, since we have little idea of what goods ought to direct the kind of experimentation we should support.

This issue becomes particularly troublesome when dealing with experimentation on children, and some normative account of parental responsibility seems unavoidable.

Chapters 7 and 8 are also important, because they were written at the request of government ethics committees who had the responsibility of recommending government policy regarding experimentation on children and *in-vitro* fertilization. I hope that these essays will counter the often-made criticism that anyone who attempts to think theologically about such issues has no contribution to make to the public debate. What I had to say to these committees may not have been what they wanted to hear, but I hope that by arguing as I did they were helped to see the issues from another perspective. I certainly think Christians have a duty to make a contribution to the public debates of this country, and I do not see how we can do so by compromising what we have to say at the beginning in the interest of not offending the pluralistic consensus.

The last section of this book is the most clearly defined by the subject matter with which the chapters deal — namely, the mentally handicapped. I was hesitant to group these essays together in this way, as I feared it would only reinforce those assumptions that underwrite the ghettoization of the mentally handicapped. However I think the reader will discover that the moral issues raised by the mentally retarded are almost the same as those entailed by our commitment to care for the sick through the agency of medicine. In particular, questions of the nature and place of suffering cannot be avoided. Thus in many ways this section of the book is crucial for the full expression of the position I have staked out in the first two parts.

The primary argument of this book, put in its simplest terms, is that a humane medicine is impossible to sustain in a society which lacks the moral capacity to care for the mentally handicapped. Moreover the "care" provided must be governed by a regard and respect for the mentally handicapped as people who exist for reasons other than simply being the recipients of our care. Only when a society is capable of supporting and sustaining that sense of care does it have the moral capacity to be peaceable. That, of course, is finally why I am so doubtful that the ethos of freedom that Engelhardt thinks necessary for assuring a peaceable community is in fact capable of doing so. For such an ethos is incapable of giving any reason why, as a society, we should be willing to care for and be with the mentally handicapped. Thus what appears to be a book about medicine turns out really to be book about social and political theory. I hope that will not seem odd to those who have graciously taken the time to read through these essays.

NOTES

1. Verhey's article nicely documents the ways Christians felt it necessary to transform the oath before they could swear it. As I try to show in chapter 2, medicine is shaped by what I call the "wisdom of the body" that in a certain sense is a "natural morality." Yet the "natural" is not known except through the development of a tradition that enables such wisdom to be passed from one generation to another. In some ways the development of "scientific medicine," which in so many ways is to be welcomed, can give the illusion that medicine no longer needs to rely on such wisdom.

2. This article is but a short overview of Engelhardt's forthcoming book, *Bioethics: An Introduction and Critique.*

3. I am certainly not opposed to contraception, but I think that the moral questions raised by contraception have not been sufficiently thought through by our culture. Ironically the Roman Catholic condemnation of contraception has prevented the kind of moral reflection we need if we are to rightly think through the issues raised by contraception. For by appealing to the "nature" of intercourse in an effort to show why every act of sexual intercourse must be open to conception, the question of why we ought to be open to having children at all has not been discussed.

REFERENCES

[1] Engelhardt, H. Tristram. 1982. "Bioethics in Pluralist Societies," *Perspectives in Biology and Medicine* 26, no. 1: 64–77.

[2] Toulmin, Stephen. 1982. "How Medicine Saved the Life of Ethics," *Perspectives in Biology and Medicine* 25, no. 4: 736–750.

[3] Verhey, Allen. 1984. "The Doctor's Oath — and a Christian Swearing it." In *Respect and Care in Medical Ethics*, ed. David Smith. New York: University Press of America.

PART ONE

Medicine as a Moral Art

1

Reflections on Suffering, Death, and Medicine

Mortality, Medicine, and Suffering

This essay is an attempt to sort out some of the issues involved in the assumption that the task of medicine is to relieve suffering. This is a common and powerful assumption, but I think we will find that on analysis it is not as straightforwardly clear as we assume. Moreover, by investigating this question I hope to throw some light on why medicine is best understood as a moral art.

I began to think about the meaning and status of suffering in relation to medicine when I encountered a case in the neonatal ward at a large hospital. A baby was allowed to die before an adequate diagnosis could be made because the mother did not want the child. I noticed that many people involved in the case justified the decision to let the baby die, which involved taking the infant off the respirator, on grounds that even if the child had been cared for, all it had to look forward to was a lifetime of physical and mental suffering. I assume they meant that the child would have to deal with severe physical problems and ugliness, in addition to having an unwilling mother.

I am not interested in trying to analyze whether the decision in that case was right or not, but what interested me was the idea that it was better for the child to die rather than experience a life of suffering. I suspect many feel the same way about spina-bifida children — thus we say they mercifully or even happily died. We seem to assume that when children will have only a life of suffering it is better that they die young.

However, the more I thought about it the more I began to think there is something odd about our sense that death is better than a life of suffering. I wrote an essay suggesting that the alleged obligation of doctors to eliminate suffering cannot be understood to be unqualified.[1] This is so not only because we know that therapy can require us to endure suffering, but also and more importantly because it seems odd that in the name of eliminating suffering, we eliminate the sufferer.

Moreover, the idea that a child might be allowed to die in order to spare it a life of suffering is inconsistent with our usual approach to the suffering which we inevitably experience as a part of life. The only difference is in kind, degree, and time. The problem is that most of us are unlucky enough to be born without any disease or handicap which would allow our parents to let us die.

It seems, therefore, that if one of the aims of medicine is to eliminate suffering it surely must be a highly qualified aim. The kind of qualification, however, remains vague. To understand this we have to raise the following extremely confusing question: What is suffering? What is its relationship to pain? How are suffering and death related? I suspect that such questions may be as unanswerable as they are important, but I am going to try to make some headway on them.

I do this partly because I think the question of suffering and its elimination may be one of the most fruitful avenues through which the relation between Christian convictions and medical practice can be explored. I want to at least raise the possibility that the most decisive challenge which medicine raises for Christian convictions and morality involves the attempt to make suffering pointless and thus subject to elimination. I am not sure whether or not it stems from my Christian or Southern roots, but I have always thought it odd that anyone should think it possible or even a good thing to eliminate all suffering. Suffering, I have been taught, is not something you eliminate, but rather something with which you must learn to live. Will Campbell suggests this in his autobiography, which depicts what it means to grow up in the South in hard times. "I do not recall our being happy. A family of six, living on a small cotton farm during the depression, growing no more than five or six bales of cotton a year which sold for a few cents a pound, did not think in those terms. Even married couples did not think in those terms. Happiness was not something promised. Happiness was not part of the contract. If it came, we experienced it without naming it. If it didn't, we couldn't complain, not aware that we were due it or that it ever existed."[2]

This point, however, can be put in a less biographical way. As Alasdair MacIntyre has asserted: "Any account of morality which does not allow for the fact that my death may be required of me at any moment is an inadequate account"[3] — an assertion that is perhaps too dramatic, but one I take to be correct. But if it is correct, then it is equally true that no account of the moral life which is worthy of our serious consideration can avoid asking us to endure suffering. Indeed, the morally interesting question is not whether we are asked to suffer, but how and for what we are asked to suffer.

It is important to note that MacIntyre's point is not that suffering is necessarily connected with morality because it is impossible to avoid, but rather that it is impossible to avoid in the context of our moral convictions. Suffering is not morally significant only because things happen to us that we cannot avoid, but because the demands of morality cannot be satisfied without asking the self to submit to limits imposed by morality itself. In this sense, without allowing ourselves and others to suffer we could not be human or humane.

This is not intuitively obvious, however, since we generally think that suffering of all kinds should be avoided. To see the value of suffering we only have to ask what we would think of anyone who did not have the capacity to suffer (including God). Such a person could not bear grief or misfortune, and thus would in effect give up the capacity to be human (or divine). For it is our capacity to feel grief and to identify with the misfortune of others which is the basis for our ability to recognize our fellow humanity. Colin Turnbull notes in *The Mountain People* that the Ik argued, "Who knows what the other is feeling? In fact you only know your own feeling."[4] As a result Turnbull lost the ability to regard these tragically damaged people as fellow human sufferers, just as they lost the ability to experience joy with another. It seems that our ability to feel joy is correlative to our willingness to be open to the suffering of another.

In that respect it is useful to reflect on our reaction to someone suffering: suffering makes the other a stranger and our first reaction is to be repelled. Suffering makes people's otherness stand out in strong relief, but that otherness is exactly the condition necessary to force recognition of them and of ourselves. For example, I suspect that one of the problems with suffering is that it alienates us from ourselves — "this thing that is happening to me is not me." But it is exactly the ability to make the suffering mine that is crucial if I am to be an integral self.

I suspect that it is only when this is recognized that we can begin to understand why medicine is a moral art. It is the burden of those who care for the suffering to know how to teach the suffering that they are not thereby excluded from the human community. In this sense medicine's primary role is to bind the suffering and the nonsuffering into the same community. Unfortunately, medicine is used too often to guard us from those who suffer.

But it is hard to say these things without being misunderstood. I am not saying that we ought to welcome suffering. We certainly ought not to enjoy suffering and we rightly think that anyone who does must be pathological, for that is our attitude toward masochism. Suffering should not be sought, but it ought to be accepted, at least in certain forms.

Nor do I want to claim that suffering ought to be accepted because by doing so we will be better people. Suffering is seldom a school for character, but rather a test for character. It may reveal us as better or worse than we had thought ourselves to be. Suffering can just as easily destroy us as it can make us more resolute. Suffering cannot be justified therefore because it may provide us with an occasion to grow. Indeed, as Iris Murdoch is fond of pointing out through her novels, suffering is seldom ennobling, because it takes an extraordinary person to survive either great suffering or happiness. My point, however, is that even if suffering is destructive in particular instances, the destruction is still a sign of strength as our pledge as humankind that we continue to be willing to risk caring.

Now if that is true, then the question remains as to what is the relation between morality and medicine in the light of the commitment of the latter to prevent suffering and death. Are medicine and morality inextricably at odds? That we can ask such a question should be a clue that we have put the issue too crudely. For we must be using a far too uncritical sense of "suffering." Surely we should be able to distinguish between different kinds of suffering? Or even more importantly, we should be able to distinguish the descriptive question of what suffering is from the normative question or whether suffering is good or bad. Then we would be able to make discriminating judgments about what kinds of suffering are good and under what conditions it is appropriate to try to alleviate it. What medicine tries to do is not to eliminate suffering and death, but unnecessary suffering and untimely death.

But how are we to know what is to count for unnecessary and

untimely? That such an issue is not as straightforward as it seems can be illustrated by the fact that even though we assume it is a good thing to avoid unnecessary suffering, I suspect it would be very hard to survive morally a life devoid of unnecessary suffering.[5] For the arbitrariness which we associate with the word "unnecessary" seems to be an essential element in learning to act morally in a world in which our moral convictions may well make us more vulnerable to the unexpected.

Nor am I sure that it is very helpful to distinguish between physical pain and suffering.[6] The force of such a distinction would be to associate medical care with pain, but the problem with that is that pain is inextricably subjective. That does not mean that pain is always a form of suffering, since we do not think it odd to say that someone is in pain and yet deny they are suffering. But the first person character of such avowals is a clue that pain is also not easily distinguished from suffering, for obviously pain can cause us to suffer.[7]

Boeyink is on the right track when he suggests that we "ordinarily mean by suffering an anguish which we experience, not only as a pressure to change, but as a threat to our composure, our integrity, and the fulfillment of our intentions."[8] But if this is the case, then it is not at all clear that we will be able to distinguish as clearly as we might like between the descriptive question of what suffering is and its evaluative force. For it seems that what distinguishes suffering from pain is suffering's personal quality.

It may rightly be objected that pain is often very personal. And even if we associate suffering with that which strikes at the self, intense pain can certainly do that. It makes us not ourselves, and no doubt one of the functions of medicine is to deal with that kind of suffering. Put paradoxically, it may be that the function of medicine is to relieve painful suffering which makes it impossible for us to claim suffering as our own. And the only one who can tell us when we are suffering that kind of pain is the agent.

Conceptual Forays into Suffering

But what I have been doing so far should be the occasion for a good deal of rustling in the philosophical backbenches. This kind of general reflection cannot get us anywhere, for what is needed is some hard conceptual analysis. I could not agree more, but I want to warn you that we cannot expect too much of such analysis. We can perhaps say a little more clearly what we mean by suffering and how it relates to pain and death, but I think we will find that the inexorably personal or, as I would prefer, interpretative character of suffering will defy neat analysis.

We assume that suffering is a natural category—after all we all have had the experience of suffering. But our assumption that we have had a common experience of suffering is misleading, for no one simply suffers. One always suffers from something. Our ability to recognize our suffering means that suffering always takes place in an interpretative context. In a sense, therefore, we must be taught that and how we suffer. That such is the case, however, does not prevent us from characterizing the general nature of suffering, as long as we remember that in fact we do not suffer in general, but from this or that in this or that way.

Suffering has as its root sense the idea of submitting or being forced to submit to and endure some particular set of circumstances. H. R. Niebuhr says, "Because suffering is the exhibition of the presence in our existence of that which is not under our control, or of the intrusion into our self-legislating existence of an activity operating under another law than ours, it cannot be brought adequately within spheres of teleological or deontological ethics. Yet it is in response to suffering that many and perhaps all men . . . define themselves, take on character, develop their ethos."[9] Thus we usually think of the sufferer as being a victim or patient.

However, we should be careful not to attribute a completely passive meaning to suffering as we also use the word to mean endure, hold out, resist, or to sustain. Thus we say "he suffered in silence," or that some people suffer fools gladly and others not at all. These examples suggest that suffering combines a peculiar passivity with a sense of agency. Some forms of suffering involve more passivity and others involve more agency.

In the medical context, however, the passive aspect of suffering seems to dominate. Perhaps this is why we think that there may be a necessary connection between suffering and death, since we tend to think of death as that in which we are most passive (although that may not be so). Louis Lavelle states something along this line: "The strongest bonds uniting one with life stand out nakedly as soon as they are endangered, as soon as they reach a breaking point. Suffering is a threat. Even in its most elementary form there is an evocation of death, the idea of a transition from life to death."[10] On this view each act of suffering is but an intimation of the ultimate act of suffering — i.e., death.

But I remain unconvinced that every form of suffering is an intimation of death. It may be correct that death is the ultimate form of suffering (we can "suffer death"), but I am not sure that this means or counts for much. At the very least it seems that such a claim is empirically false, since many see death as a release from suffering. Of course it may be replied that this is but to balance one form of suffering against another. That may be, but if so it seems to me that we are close to losing any sense of suffering. It becomes a word to describe life itself, rather than a word to redescribe what is inextricably bound up with living.

For all life is made up of "what is done to us." If suffering is simply a word for life, then it does not seem to have much sense. It is a little like some Christians who want to describe everything — the next breath we inhale, the confrontation with another, our sense of self — as manifestations of God's grace. If God's grace is everything, then it is not very interesting, because there is nothing in particular with which it can be associated.

To deny suffering a general meaning does not mean that we must be able to provide an analysis of the conceptual boundaries of suffering. However, after trying to read all I could get my hands on concerning the meaning of suffering, I am convinced that never has there been a word used with such an uncritical assumption that everyone knows what they are talking about. For example, in David Bakan's *Disease, Pain and Sacrifice: Toward a Psychology of Suffering*, we are never offered even in the most cursory fashion what he means by suffering.[11] Rather, suffering is claimed to be a correlative of "telic decentralization." Bakan uses this phrase as a way to claim that suffering has biological, psychological, and existential roots. While this may be a helpful reminder that suffering is a threat to our biological and personal integrity, it does little to help us see how these two senses of integrity may be related.

Perhaps the absence of the kind of analysis about suffering we desire tells us something about the grammar of the word — namely, that any use of the notion of suffering is context dependent. Our assumption that suffering is a universal phenomenon makes us forget that we can only talk intelligently about it through the use of paradigm instances. In other words, the meaning of suffering varies from one interpretative context to another. As a result, suffering as a moral notion is often used equivocally because we forget that it can only be used analogically.

In terms of the analysis Kovesi offers of the word "good,"[12] suffering is an open notion and therefore we cannot and should not expect it to do much moral work. It can mean anything from an absence of happiness to enduring extreme pain, and there is no way to prefer one usage to another on conceptual grounds. Any attempt to distinguish various forms of suffering and their value therefore depends on a normative argument which must make appeal to ways of life which are thought to be admirable. For example, we rightly think that anyone who contracts malaria or suffers from Huntington's disease should be cared for, but what we forget is that such a commitment often embodies the moral assumption that such "suffering" is pointless and thus, if possible, should be eliminated.

I suspect that the temptation in medicine is to try to restrict the meaning of suffering to a biological context in the interest of protecting medicine from being used as a tool to alleviate every form of suffering. For it seems that the closer suffering is to "pain," the more objective it is and therefore the less dependent it is on an interpretative context, or to be precise, the more the interpretative context presupposes a widely shared agreement that this is the kind of suffering that is unnecessary and that therefore ought to be alleviated. Such a suggestion has much to commend it, but I have called it a temptation because it can lead us both socially and individually to have unrealistic attitudes about the identification and disvalue of suffering.

Does Suffering Have a Point?

But the view I have taken so far may fail entirely to deal with why suffering bothers us so deeply and is so hard to analyze—namely, the idea that suffering has no point. For example, I suggested above that medicine is probably best thought of as trying to alleviate unnecessary suffering, but it is at least reasonable to suggest that the very character of all suffering is unnecessary. If that is the case, there is no point in enduring suffering except as a way of expressing our irrational desire to go on living.

The idea that suffering has no point is so threatening to us that we are hardly even able to contemplate, much less embody, the implications of such a view. As Paul Claudel suggests, "Happy is he who suffers and who knows why." I suspect that as much as one might intellectually reject the suggestion made by some Christians that our suffering, including our suffering from disease, is the appropriate punishment for our sins, we continue to accept much of our suffering in terms of some crude sense of desert. For it seems infinitely preferable to suffer for a wrong, even if we think the suffering is inappropriate to the wrong, than to suffer for no reason. From this perspective, the Christian notion of sin turns out to be a remarkably comforting notion. Moreover, I suspect that it would be a mistake to disassociate entirely the relation of sin and suffering since sin is no more a natural category than suffering. Just as we must be taught to sin, so we must be taught to suffer for the right things and for failing to do the right things. Otherwise, suffering is a far too meaningless phenomenon.

There is moreover the problem of whether it is possible conceptually to grasp the idea of pointless suffering (though of course we may in certain instances be able to think that a certain form of suffering is pointless). For if suffering to be recognized, i.e., named, involves an interpretative context, then the very interpretation seems to carry a "point." The interpretation at least places the suffering in a narrative context even if the narrative is thought to be absurdist. I am not suggesting that explanation carries with it a justification, but only that the explanation at least lets us claim the suffering as ours. Thus every doctor can testify to the importance of indicating the causes of suffering (even if it is cancer) because the patient, knowing the cause of his suffering, is comforted by being able to name his affliction. Somehow it domesticates suffering if we are able to locate it within our world.

Christian convictions are interesting in this regard as Christians, drawing on the life of Jesus, tend to make the very pointlessness of suffering morally significant. As Bakan suggests, the cross has provided a psychologically powerful means for many to overcome the essential loneliness and privacy of pain.[13] The cross provides a pattern of interpretation which allows one to locate the pointlessness of suffering within a cosmic framework.

It should be noted, however, that the association of the cross with human suffering has often perverted the Christian life. Not only does it encourage some unwisely to accept avoidable suffering, but from

a theological point of view it makes us think all our suffering is akin
to Christ's. But suffering or even self-sacrifice is not a virtue for Christians when that suffering or sacrifice is not formed by Christ's cross.
And that cross

> was not an inexplicable or chance event, which happened to strike him,
> like illness or accident. To accept the cross as his destiny, to move toward
> it and even to provide it, when he could well have done otherwise, was
> Jesus' constantly reiterated free choice; and he warns his disciples lest
> their embarking on the same path be less conscious of its costs (Luke
> 14:25–33). The cross of Calvary was not a difficult family situation, not
> a frustration of visions of personal fulfillment, a crushing debt or nag-
> ging in-law; it was the political, legally to be expected result of a moral
> clash with the powers ruling his society. Already the early Christians
> had to be warned against claiming merit for any and all suffering; only
> if their suffering be innocent, and a result of the evil will of their adver-
> saries, may it be understood as meaningful before God.[14]

When Christians try to explain all suffering in and of itself having
theological significance we end up vacating the cross of its significance
because we fail to remember that what is important about the cross
is who was crucified there. Moreover such accounts of suffering tempt
us to masochistic accounts of the Christian life that cannot help but
belie the joy characteristic of the Christian orientation.

Thus in I Peter 3:14–18 we read

> But even if you do suffer for righteousness sake, you will be blessed.
> Have no fear of them, nor be troubled, but in your hearts reverence
> Christ as Lord. Always be prepared to make a defense to any one who
> calls you to account for the hope that is in you, yet do it with gentleness
> and reverence; and keep your conscience clear, so that when you are
> abused, those who revile your good behavior in Christ may be put to
> shame. For it is better to suffer for doing right, if that should be God's
> will, than for doing wrong. For Christ also died for sins once for all,
> the righteous for the unrighteous, that he might bring us to God, be-
> ing put to death in the flesh but made alive in the spirit.

It seems to me that the logic of the Christian identification of
and value of suffering may indicate a general point about what it means
to say that suffering has no point. For the point that some suffering
lacks is that it serves no purpose in our moral project. One assumes

that a great deal of illness has this character, though the suffering may be necessary if the agent is to know how to integrate illness into his or her project.

From this perspective, medicine can be interpreted as the attempt to have us view our suffering as pointless, thus making it subject to therapeutic intervention. In other words, medicine tends to break the moral link between our suffering and our projects by suggesting that our suffering is pointless. Medicine thus schools us to think of suffering in terms of a mechanical model. This is often done in the name of science — we now know that cancer is caused by X or Y and not by living a sinful life. But what we must understand is that "science" so used is motivated by the powerful moral claim that our suffering should not be brought within the realm of moral intentionality.

If the analysis above has been correct, however, it can be asked if there is hope for this strategy to succeed. Even stronger, it might be asked if such a strategy is not finally self-deceptive. For the recognition of suffering is inextricably moral; that is, if we think that some of our suffering is a proper punishment or a necessary result of our convictions, what we suffer and what we have done is in close relationship. From such a moral perspective the kind of suffering medicine seeks to alleviate is that in which there is no connection between the kind of suffering and our project. But then what are we to do with the claim of some that we fail to live up to our moral potential when we fail to claim all forms of suffering — even the pointless disease and pain — as our own? We might at least consider the possibility that the reason medicine has so much power over our lives is because we have too willingly assumed that suffering is pointless.

To reclaim the moral meaning of suffering does not mean, however, that we must be committed to denying the intervention of medicine to relieve suffering. There is nothing incompatible in understanding our suffering as contributing in some manner to our moral project, but thinking that such suffering should be alleviated if possible. What it may require is that we learn to understand in a different manner what we are doing when we intervene medically to remove suffering.

Perhaps more interesting, however, is how this view of suffering may require us to rethink what we mean by autonomy. Suffering is often regarded as a threat to autonomy, but if I have been right, we only gain autonomy by our willingness to make suffering our own through its incorporation into our moral projects. For autonomy is a correlative of our having a narrative through which we can make our suffering our own.[15] Insofar as medicine denies us our suffering, rather than being a way to regain autonomy, it can be a threat or temptation to lose our autonomy.

Suffering, Death, and Life Choices

As a means of making this analysis less abstract, I will try to respond briefly to some of the hard cases which involve a choice between death and continuing to suffer. It is important to note, however, that my remarks are not meant to entail that people should be prevented from dying when they wish. Rather, I am concerned with how an agent should live out his or her life in suffering. But even from that perspective, I am not at all sure it is helpful to characterize these kinds of choices as involving a balancing of suffering and death.

Take for example the case of someone facing a choice between staying on dialysis, which will enable a life of suffering to be sustained, and having a transplant, which will provide freedom from suffering but shorten life. I have tried to analyze this choice in terms of balancing suffering and death, and getting nowhere I finally resorted to asking myself what I would do. It occurred to me that what I would do had almost nothing to do with balancing suffering against death. I would take the transplant if by doing so I could continue to do the kinds of things I would like to do. To put such decisions in terms of balancing suffering against death rightly seems bizarre. For such a decision is not made in terms of such balancing at all, because suffering fits into the narrative of one's life and is thus not the kind of thing you can calculate.

What about those cases, however, in which we have to choose for another to undergo treatment which will entail suffering? Again, I think the issue really cannot turn on the extent of the suffering, for it is odd to choose death for someone in the name of sparing them suffering. Rather, I think that we must be careful not to rob others of the necessary means to be human in our attempt to spare their suffering. I do not think we can or should will a world without suffering, and the question is whether in allowing the suffering to die we are actually removing our own suffering. As Claudel says "One's own sorrow is nothing, but the sorrow one has caused to others makes bitter the bread in the mouth."

Children make particularly hard cases in this respect; some children have to suffer and we have to allow them to suffer. We would be disrespectful of them if we always assumed that they were unable to deal with their suffering. The lives of children suffering from leukemia provide a particularly striking example of this.

Moreover, we need to maintain sufficient motivation to try to deal with the basis of their distress. I suspect childhood suffering is so hard partly because it is so difficult to be helpless in the face of it. Our very humanity cries out for its elimination. But I suspect that we must learn how to be patient and endure the suffering with them. Such patience is at the heart of medical care.

Again I wonder if the cases at the level of social policy really turn on being able to provide a cost/benefit formula comparing suffering to death. For example, it is clear that arthritis research should be funded more, but that is not because I think we should prefer to stop the suffering of the living at the cost of the death of others. Rather, it has to do with the ends of medicine. If the end of medicine is health rather than the prevention of death, then obviously arthritis is an extremely debilitating disease for our health.

Christianity and Medicine

If the above analysis has been right, then the idea that we can balance or calculate how much suffering is preferable to death, in order to make medical decisions, is a mistake. Rather our decisions must turn on what we think our lives are for, and not how much suffering they contain or how long we can avoid death. But to put the question in this context is a reminder that medicine as a moral art depends for its direction on profound convictions drawn from a more morally inclusive community.

For example, contemporary medicine is often criticized for trying to keep people alive beyond all reason. And it is certainly the case that too often people are subjected to medical intervention that only prolongs death rather than offering any way to return to health. However, the distinction between prolonging death and returning to health is not self-evident. To know the difference between prolonging death and returning to health is correlative to a community's understanding of how health contributes to appropriate life projects. In the absence of any agreed upon sense of health as a moral notion, our culture has tended to make the prevention of death the overriding norm to inform medical practice. As a result we try to transform what are essentially moral decisions into calculations about trade-offs between suffering and death. But, as we have seen, suffering and death defy quantification.

If medical care is to find a way out of this dilemma it will depend on our ability to reclaim medicine as a moral activity at the service of a community's moral projects. It is in the context of such a task that it makes sense to think that there might be something like a Christian medicine. For as I have tried to argue elsewhere, it is by no means clear that Christians share the same attitudes as non-Christians concerning the preservation of life.[16] We do not believe that life is an end in itself. Rather we regard life as a gift that provides the means for service; not the least of which is our willingness to stay alive amid the ambiguity and destructiveness of our existence. We thus see the very existence of another as a testimony and support that we too can go on living in a hopeful and trustful manner.

Therefore, we do not believe it is appropriate to seek our death as a relief from suffering. For the very willingness to carry suffering is but a continuation of the kind of moral commitment that has sustained our lives together in the first place. At the same time, however, Christians do not believe that life must be preserved at all costs. As a result it is incumbent on us to develop expectations among ourselves when it is appropriate to fight death no more. The corresponding form of medical care we might well find would not only be more worthy and appropriate of Christian convictions, but might also result in helping those who do not share our convictions to find appropriate ways to fight and accept death.

NOTES

1. S. Hauerwas, "Suffering, Medical Ethics, and the Retarded Child," in *Truthfulness and Tragedy* (Notre Dame, Ind.: University of Notre Dame Press, 1977), pp. 164–168.

2. W. Campbell, *Brother to a Dragonfly* (New York: Seabury Press, 1978).

3. A. MacIntyre, "Can Medicine Dispense with a Theological Perspective on Human Nature?" in *Knowledge, Value, and Belief*, ed. Engelhardt and Callahan (Hastings-on-Hudson, N.Y.: The Hastings Center, 1977), pp. 26-27.

4. C. Turnbull, *The Mountain People* (New York: Simon and Schuster, 1972), p. 253.

5. The lack of any attempt to deal with "luck" as integral to the moral life is one of the greatest deficiencies of contemporary moral philosophy. However, see Bernard Williams, *Moral Luck* (Cambridge: Cambridge University Press, 1981). Nozick's criticisms of Rawls are also interesting in this respect. See *Anarchy, State, and Utopia* (New York: Basic Books, 1974), pp. 213-216.

6. D. Boeyink, "Pain and Suffering," *Journal of Religious Ethics* 2 (1974): 85-98.

7. L. McCollough, "Pain, Suffering, and Life-Extending Technologies," unpublished paper for Death and Dying Group, Hastings Center for Society, Ethics, and the Life Sciences.

8. Boeyink, p. 86.

9. H. R. Niebuhr, *The Responsible Self* (New York: Harper and Row, 1963), p. 60.

10. L. Lavelle, *Evil and Suffering* (New York: Macmillan, 1963), pp. 59-60.

11. D. Bakan, *Disease, Pain, and Sacrifice: Toward a Psychology of Suffering* (Boston: Beacon Press, 1968).

12. J. Kovesi, *Moral Notions* (New York: Humanities Press, 1967).

13. Bakan, pp. 64–65.

14. J. H. Yoder, *The Politics of Jesus* (Grand Rapids, Mich.: Eerdmans, 1972), p. 132.

15. See for example Part I of *Truthfulness and Tragedy*. For example Stanley Cavell suggests that suffering and tragedy are the necessary conditions for us to be able to act at all. The purpose of tragedy "is not to purge us of pity and terror, but to make us capable of feeling them again, and this means showing us that there is a place to act upon them. This does not mean that tragedy now must become political. Because it was always political, always about the incompatibility between a particular love and a particular social arrangement for love" (p. 347). He locates the root of tragedy and suffering in the self's necessity of identity. Thus the source of tragedy in the past was that people could only find out who they were by finding themselves the cause of tragedy. "They are heroic because they care completely who they are; they are tragic because what they find is incompatible with their existence. Our tragic fact is that we find ourselves at the cause of tragedy, but without finding ourselves. . . . In the typical situation of tragic heroes, time and space converge to a point at which an ultimate care is exposed and action must be taken which impales one's life upon the founding care of that life. . . .

Death, so caused, may be mysterious, but what founds these lives is clear enough: the capacity to love, the strength to found a life upon a love. That the love becomes incompatible with that life is tragic, but that it is maintained until the end is heroic. People capable of such love could have removed mountains; instead it has caved in upon them. One moral of such events is obvious: if you would avoid tragedy [and suffering], avoid love; if you cannot avoid love, avoid integrity; if you cannot avoid integrity, avoid the world; if you cannot avoid the world, destroy it. Our tragedy differs from this classical chain not in its conclusion but in the fact that the conclusion has been reached without passing through love, in the fact that no love seems worth founding one's life upon, or that society—and therefore I myself— can allow no context in which love, for anything but itself, can be expressed . . . . Our problem, in getting back to beginnings, will not be to find the thing we have always cared about, but to discover whether we have it in us always to care about something." S. Cavell, *Must We Mean What We Say?* (New York: Scribner's, 1969), pp. 349–350.

16. S. Hauerwas, *Vision and Virtue* (Notre Dame, Ind.: University of Notre Dame Press, rpt. 1981), pp. 166-186.

2

Authority and the Profession
of Medicine

Authority and Medicine: Some General Considerations

Both medicine and religion are systems of authority. It is not surprising that there should be conflict between them, as each cannot but help to claim some of the other's territory. For many religious thinkers the current supremacy of medicine's authority provides a tempting target in their efforts to reclaim some of their own past glory. Thus theologians underwrite claims of patient autonomy in an effort to humble the authority of physicians. It is my thesis that such a strategy not only will not work, but fails to illumine how, religiously, we ought to regard medicine's rightful claims to authority. Therefore I will try to offer a constructive account of authority, and in particular the authority of medicine, that will avoid the crude alternatives of assuming we must choose between autonomy or paternalism.

The lack of an adequate philosophical account of authority certainly contributes to the confusion of so complex a topic. Although sociologists like to refer to Max Weber's famous distinction between charismatic, traditional, and legal-rational authority [19], this typology fails to clarify what it means to acknowledge an authority as legitimate.[1] Authority is fundamentally a political-moral concept; therefore, its meaning is dependent upon an understanding of the nature of human community and the moral good. In this regard, Alasdair MacIntyre argues that the lack of consensus concerning the latter makes it impossible to formulate an intelligible concept or practice of authority [12]. If MacIntyre is correct, it is easy to see how frustrating it can be to address the subject of authority in the practice of medicine.[2]

In spite of confusion regarding the general question of authority in our society, medicine actually may be able to provide some insight into the concept of authority. For medicine does seem to be one of

39

the few areas of modern life where some sense of authority remains viable. It is important to recognize, for example, that MacIntyre's argument turns not on the inherent character of medicine, but on society's lack of any common consensus and tradition through which the variety of goods can be ordered in a coherent manner. The problem of authority in medicine, therefore, is not peculiar to medicine, but is another indication of the general problem of authority today.[3]

There can be no doubt that physicians individually and as members of an elite profession continue to command *de facto* authority. For example, it has been one of my duties to teach seminarians who have no experience and little conception of the past power and authority of the clergy. Most assume they are entering a devalued profession in which any authority they may attain depends largely on their personal characteristics. To help them at least understand the authority of the clergy as role and office, I call their attention to how they regard their physicians. By revealing their willingness to accept direction from their physicians even when they often know little about the basis for such advice, I try to give them a sense of how people once looked to clergymen for direction. By its very nature, then, authority seems to involve people's willingness to accept the judgments of another as superior to their own on the basis of that person's office and assumed skills ([12], p. 200).

A number of people might argue with the choice of such a parallel, especially if they infer incorrectly that clergymen should behave like physicians. From their perspective there could be no poorer paradigm than medicine for providing a resource for rethinking the nature of authority. This contention is based on the charge that reliance on physicians is justified neither morally or medically. When patients give such power to physicians, poor medical care results, because they are robbed of their own resources to maintain health. Attributing such authority to physicians encourages a medical authoritarianism and cultivates an almost uncontrolled resentment against the medical profession in general.

Although physicians may still be able to command *de facto* authority, many would question if such authority is legitimate, since it seems antithetical to our society's stress on autonomy. Why, then, have physicians individually and as a group been able to continue to command such authority in spite of what seems to be a widespread dissatisfaction with them? It is a singularly interesting question. Richard

Blum notes that the "average citizen places the medical profession and its members at the top rung of social prestige."[4] While prestige is not the same as authority, it does suggest the level of respect that contributes to the authority of the profession of medicine. Physicians are perceived by the majority to possess a particular moral commitment and special expertise by which they perform an irreplaceable service — to make people well when they become ill. Herein lies the contrast with the loss of authority in the clergy: People are rather unsure whether they need saving, but they are certain that they want to get well when they are ill.

The critic of the authority and power of medicine may well respond that this contrast is exactly the point. For the authority of the physician is morally suspect *because* it derives from and exploits fears of illness and humankind's hopeless attempts to avoid death. Authority attributed to medicine (an attribution made all the more compelling by medicine's often exaggerated claims of being a science) is based on false and self-deceiving presuppositions of the power of medicine to cure. Though patients are the ones who confer such power on medicine, physicians are morally culpable for reinforcing, if not positively encouraging, such mistaken attitudes. The very illnesses that drive people to seek aid in the first place are used unfairly by physicians to reinforce their unjustified power over patients' lives. Rather than offering a defensible paradigm of authority, such critics would say, medicine remains one of the last institutions thwarting the individual's claim to rightful autonomy against all illegitimate authorities of the past.

Yet the authority of physicians shows no signs of crumbling. If those who approach these issues from a sociology of knowledge perspective are even close to being right, physicians are in an impregnable position. In fact, if physicians ever run short of disease or illnesses, it seems they are capable of helping to discover new ones. In this way, the necessity of physicians' services is assured, as well as the necessity of remaining under their authority.[5] Moreover, it is alleged, the moral commitments that physicians use to underwrite the autonomy of their profession are yet another way of increasing illegitimate power over patients.[6]

It is important to note, however, that a number of these attacks on medicine draw on a political philosophy which presupposes that the autonomy of the individual renders all relations that are less than fully "voluntary" morally problematic.[7] Hence, all claims of authority are suspect. Insofar as illness is perceived to be a coercive condition, the power of physicians cannot help but be seen as illegitimate and a source of continued resentment. It seems, therefore, that the task must be to make the physician-patient relationship conform as nearly as possible to a contract between two voluntary agents.

Such an ideal, however, not only distorts the kind of relationship that should and often does evolve between physician and patient, but it assumes a false political and ethical ideal for all human relations. In contrast, in this essay the claim is that medicine *does* offer an alternative conception and practice of authority that can help us to appreciate how other forms of authority should function in morally healthy societies.[8] To be sure, physicians often misunderstand and abuse their authority, but this is not sufficient reason for denying them all authority. Instead, it is more desirable to try to understand the sense in which the authority exercised by physicians is valid.

Part of the difficulty of trying to develop a constructive account of medical authority is that the dominant moral and political conceptions of authority in our society make it hard to acknowledge the different kinds of authority that still function in some social institutions. Richard Sennett has observed that the current dilemma of authority is that people feel attracted to strong figures whose power is not considered to be illegitimate. They try to protect themselves by denying authority to these figures or, even more self-deceptively, by claiming that no one (not even these strong figures) has power over them ([16], p. 26). Those forms of authority which people find in their lives, moreover, appear destructive, because they appear to serve any good that legitimate forms of authority involve. It is important, therefore, to try to elicit a sense of how authority, and in particular authority in medicine, can function legitimately.

Authority in a Liberal Society: MacIntyre's Challenge

An account of authority that may prove helpful in understanding the authority in and of medicine is that presented in MacIntyre's "Patients as Agents" [12]. MacIntyre's essay may seem to be an odd choice, since the thrust of his argument is that it is no longer possible to provide an intelligible account of medical authority. He concludes that patients must become "agents" — as nearly as possible autonomous, since they have no other alternative. Interestingly, MacIntyre's argument is not based on a view of autonomy as a moral good, but as a last resort in a society that lacks any means of determining how goods such as life, health, and freedom are related to one another. ([12], p. 210).

Contrary to many philosophical accounts of authority, MacIntyre's does not contrast authority with rationality and/or autonomy. Indeed, he argues that authority and tradition are necessary conditions for rationality ([12], p. 201). In support of this claim he appeals to recent arguments in the philosophy of science which indicate that progress in natural science depends on the willingness of some scientists, acting on their authority, to move into areas for which there is no precedent.[9] They are able to do so because they have shown themselves as good representatives of the tradition even if now they are challenging some aspect of the tradition. That such a process is required should not be surprising, since science remains, like medicine, fundamentally a matter of judgment.[10]

The nature of this authority is very much like that of a judge in the common law tradition. For as MacIntyre points out, science as well as law are rule-governed practices in which judgments about how to understand particular cases is entrusted to certain individuals in virtue of recognition of their having experience and judgment gained through their knowledge of the tradition.[11] Such judgment is not a mechanical procedure, since it often has to go beyond existing precedents and current generalizations if it is to work out the anomalies in the tradition or meet demands of a new day. The prerequisite for the carrying on and growth of a tradition is a succession of authoritative voices. Thus, science has been able to grow because it has refused to adopt as adequate any specific methodology and instead has relied on the judgment of those skilled in the practices that constitute the scientific tradition.

According to MacIntyre, the flourishing of such a tradition and a correlative understanding of authority requires a high degree of moral consensus—that is, trust in one's fellow practitioners as well as a shared vision of the goods internal to that practice and the procedures necessary to achieve those goods. Such a consensus is also required by the very nature of the specialization needed for pursuing the particular goods within a community. Not everyone can master the same skills; specialization is encouraged because the limits of each specialist are underwritten and balanced by other community goods. Also required for the proper functioning of authority is an allocation of roles and rights within the practice and a shared acceptance of the constraints necessary to keep the practice from being distracted by external goods such as power, money, and fame ([12], pp. 201–202). (Needless to say, this is easier said than done.)

MacIntyre contends, therefore, that an authority which is internal to a *practice* is quite different from one required by an *organization*. The latter presupposes inequality of power—i.e., authority is but a name for the power that some are given to ensure compliance by others. This form of authority is necessary because an organization, in contrast to a practice, exists entirely to serve extrinsic purposes.[12] MacIntyre does not deny that often the role of authority in a practice may become so obscure that an organizational model of authority is required. It is part of the pathos of modern society that almost all forms of authority must become organizational to varying degrees.

To pursue further MacIntyre's distinction between a practice and an organization is unnecessary in the context of this paper.[13] More appropriate are some of MacIntyre's substantive, but insufficiently explicit, assumptions about community with respect to authority. The heart of his case involves an attempt to defend an account of authority that does not make the necessity of authority a correlative of human weakness. Authority is required not because human beings lack something or are innately evil. Rather, it derives from common participation in worthy endeavors. In this respect MacIntyre's basic intuitions are very similar to those of Yves Simon's account of authority [17].

Simon contends that authority originates in the plenitude of human purposes, rather than in the deficiency of human nature.[14] In contrast to political theorists such as Robert Dahl, who assumes that the problem of authority is how "to reconcile personal choice with my nature as a social being,"[15] Simon contends human nature is social exactly because community provides the means whereby the many goods people rightly desire can be actualized. Consequently, there should be a plurality of means in the pursuit of a community's common good. Indeed, the pursuit, or the conversation necessary for that pursuit, *is* in many ways the common good. For any conversation to occur a plurality is required, as well as a sufficient method of steadily procuring unity of action. Authority, therefore, is exactly that power which allows unified common action for the achievement of the common good ([17], pp. 47–48).

Authority is needed, according to Simon, because "it is desirable that particular goods should be taken care of by particular agencies" ([17], p. 72). (The diversity of skills and activities necessary for communities to flourish is a case in point.) Since those goods are not known by necessity, but must be discovered through concrete judgments, authority is essential for the pursuit of the common good. In other words, if moral and political truth were necessary or universal, there would be no need for authority. Since truth involves judgment, however, people cannot seek it unaided. Put differently, all moral goods can be known through a political process.

MacIntyre's case for authority seems to presuppose something very much like this understanding of the nature of human community. His view becomes particularly important in light of his discussion of the exercise and legitimacy of traditional medical authority. The background and practice required to make intelligible the willingness of patients to let physicians take responsibility for them — responsibility not simply in terms of advice, but responsibility that *tells* patients what they must do — involves a cultural setting in which there is a clearly established view of human good and a rational consensus on the *order* of human goods. The variety of human practices can be assigned priority in terms of the goods internal to them. Significant practices are embodied in professions which specifically pursue those goods and cultivate those virtues necessary to achieve them. For example, the goods related to rational inquiry and the virtues of intellectual honesty, self-criticism, and theoretical thinking are entrusted to the learned professions. The good of health is given to the medical profession with its concomitant virtues. There is accordingly a moral division of labor in society which requires that each part of society has trust in the other. The distribution of powers in this way is justified by the relationship of professions, goods, and virtues ([12], p. 206).

MacIntyre, like Simon, presupposes that the common good is served by "particular goods being taken care of by particular agencies." He does not assume that any society has perfectly institutionalized this pattern, but argues that something approaching this pattern has provided the basis for professions in the past, particularly medicine.[16] Only against this background can the current situation be assessed. Today in the absence of any shared moral consensus about the goods necessary for individual and community flourishing, traditional medical authority cannot be vindicated or sustained. Thus MacIntyre argues that a profession today is something anomalous:

not quite a craftsman's guild, not quite a trade union of skilled workers, not quite anything. Its various characteristics have lost their connection with the principles which made of their variety a relatively unified whole. This is what has happened in our culture, so I am suggesting, to such professions as schoolteaching and medicine, and it at once makes their peculiar claims to authority implausible and unintelligible. The recognition of authority and the concept of profession are inseparably linked.[17]

MacIntyre's account of authority aids in understanding why medicine's authority does not derive entirely from the scientific or technical skill of the physician or surgeon. The authority of the doctor is not that of the "expert," at least not in the sense in which that term is currently used.[18] Rather, a physician's authority derives from physicians' and patients' common moral beliefs and shared participation in a practice that embodies those beliefs. The physician's authority thus is based upon mastery of the moral and practical skills involved in that physician's commitment to care for and never abandon the ill and the dying. Obviously, this view involves a particular understanding of medicine which I must now try to defend.

What Medicine Professes: The Authority of the Body

To sustain the argument about the nature of authority necessitates nothing less than a philosophy of medicine that at least makes credible the claim that medicine is a practice of the kind suggested above. Edmund Pellegrino and David Thomasma have provided some insight as to what an adequate philosophy of medicine entails [15]. They reiterate that medicine is a complex activity and as such is difficult to characterize philosophically. For example, they argue that medicine is neither art nor science, but a *tertium quid* involving both but distinct from each. Medicine is the "cognitive art of applying science and persuasion through a complex human interaction in which a mutually satisfactory state of well-being is sought, and in which the uniqueness of values and disease, and the kind of institution in which care is delivered, determine the nature of the judgments made" ([15], p. 69). Or medicine is "a relation of mutual consent to effect individualized well-being by working with, and through the body" ([15], p. 80).

One aspect of Pellegrino and Thomasma's account which is crucial to any understanding of the kind of authority medicine does or at least should have is the insistence that whatever else medicine may involve, the overriding commitment of physicians is to care for individuals who come to them with complaints of illness. They conclude that "medicine *as* medicine is a process aimed at an *action* taken in the interest of a specific patient. Its chief aim is not discovery of laws of nature. The end of medicine, its justifying principle, is, in the final analysis, a moral one: the 'good' of a person seeking help" ([15], p. 147).

Pellegrino and Thomasma thus make the interesting suggestion that medicine involves not only science and art, but also virtue. They argue that what constitutes medicine is the accumulated wisdom of well-reasoned and concrete judgments about the "capacity to act with regard to the things that are good or bad for man" ([15], p. 148). The practice of medicine is thus "a habit of the mind" that embodies the good inherent in the process of healing. Since health is a good, it follows that medicine must be a virtue, because a virtue "must make right choices about the ends and purposes for which the decisions and actions are produced. Medicine must not only perform well but also act well. It must choose what should be done to heal a particular whose good is the true end of the whole activity" ([15]), p. 148).

Surely the claim that medicine is a virtue is an odd one, because a virtue is a disposition of a particular agent. Pellegrino and Thomasma, on the other hand, interpret medicine to be a relation. Of course, it is true that Aristotle called justice and friendship virtues, though each is clearly a quality of a relation rather than a good inherent to the self.[19] That a relation may be subject to virtuous formation is but a reminder that all virtues require formation through the practical judgments shaped by the wisdom of a community's tradition. Medicine, therefore, is the name for a tradition of wisdom concerning good care of the body. As such it is not a "means" to health, but rather is part of the activity of health—an activity that involves as much the participation of the patient as the physician.

Pellegrino and Thomasma's case for medicine as a moral profession goes well beyond the notion that health is a normative category.[20] The issue is not simply that medicine involves values in decisions concerning the care of particular patients, but that medicine is an activity which requires as well as enhances a virtuous life.[21] In this context, the physician is not the sole participant in the activity; rather, medicine becomes a relation that inextricably involves patient and physician. This does not mean that patients need to possess the skills of their physicians; it is sufficient that patients have moral reasons to trust physicians to support their life projects insofar as those projects involve a well-functioning body.

The very willingness of patients to permit physicians to be present as well as to lay hands on them in times of crisis is a telling indication of the physician's dependence on patients. In this respect, perhaps the best way of thinking about the medical relation is to see it as fundamentally an educational process for both doctor and patient, in which each is both teacher and learner [13]. It is from patients that physicians learn the wisdom of the body. Both physicians and patients must learn that each of them is subject to a prior authority—the authority of the body. The form and practice of medicine may change throughout history and differ from one cultural setting to another, but these differences in the end are merely reflections of different attitudes toward the body and are regulated finally by the body. Medicine thus represents a transcultural practice of learning to live with finitude.[22]

Pellegrino and Thomasma, however, properly insist that "the body" is by no means a straightforward category ([15], pp. 73–74). Each person is not simply a physical body, but a "lived body" which organizes a whole field of perceptions in addition to being the subject of a history of experience.[23] The body sets the norm for medicine because it is the "artist of its own healing" ([15], p. 79). The task of medicine is to aid that process so that individuals may better learn to live in and through their bodies, since they cannot successfully live beyond or without their bodies. Medicine is therefore a tradition of inherited wisdom and practices through which physicians acquire the responsibility to remember, learn, and pass on the skills of learning to live with a body.

As mentioned before, there is little evidence to support the claim that the health of a population is a result of the practice of medicine. Except in the case of those persons who try to justify the special privileges of medicine by this claim, its denial should not be viewed as a judgment against medicine. Those who justify privileges are responsible in part for the eventual perversion of medicine, since medical authority cannot long be sustained by promising more and more cures through technological advances.[24]

Wise physicians, on the other hand, have learned their craft better. As Eric Cassell notes, the primary task of physicians is to move the world of illness from the unknown to the known world where it can become subject to human care ([6], p. 131). Their task, however, is not limited to those who become ill. By steadfastly identifying with the ill, physicians become teachers also for the healthy. Part of the physician's vocation, therefore, is to serve as a bridge between the world of the sick and the world of the healthy.

The sick constitute a threat to us by making us aware of the frailty of our own connectedness, the thinness of our shield of reason, and the limit of our control over the world. By segregating the sick in hospitals having special rules of behavior, the threat for us and the sick is somewhat mitigated, if not entirely eliminated. It is not surprising that we do not often discuss or even secretly recognize the essential characteristics of sickness, because it would be too frightening to do so. This carries over into medicine itself. Cassell points out: "ostensibly, the physician deals only with disease elements of the illness. His manifest function is the cure of disease, but his latent function, healing, which involves restoring the sick to the world of the healthy, is a secret even to himself" ([6], p. 46). Because physicians have this task, they stand as a constant reminder that the worlds of the sick and the healthy are actually one world joined by common destiny.

Cassell provides impetus for the contention that medicine is primarily an educational process by showing how physicians act as arbitrators between patients and their bodies ([6], p. 47). Yet as important as Cassell's explicit thesis is the way in which he uses examples to make his case. For him examples help us see how he was educated by his patients to understand what medicine is about.[25] The wisdom manifest in Cassell's book is therefore a witness to the wisdom of the body that teaches "what life is really about underneath the social conventions."[26]

The point is exemplified in Cassell's observation that it is possible, and even a duty, for a physician to teach patients how to die — "to give his patients in this final stage of life the same kind of control that can be taught in earlier stages of living" ([6], p. 203). This is not to say that teaching patients how to die is the first priority. Cassell admits that the primary duty of a physician is to aid in the patient's recovery. He is not suggesting that the physician can give the patient control for which the patient does not already have the resources. Likewise, medicine should refrain from substituting technology for a patient's lack of moral resources. Physicians, however, can help their dying patient to acquire the "innate ability to command the body, and then enlist the aid of those who surround him—family, friends, and physician. Such an ability is dependent on what humans have within themselves; to that extent it is a lonely thing, as is death itself. But the dying are also dependent on others and relationship is based on trust. Both inner resources and trust in others are required, because the enemy of control is fear" ([6], p. 204).

It is ironic, though, that what people fear is not illness itself but loss of control. That fear is so all-consuming is an indication of the common misunderstanding of what control of the body entails. To control the body does not mean to "manage" or even, as Cassell suggests, to "soar" over the body ([6], p. 146), but rather to appreciate how the body's limitations are also the source of the most creative and interesting possibilities available to us.[27] By learning to live as embodied beings, that is, as people subject to disease and ultimately death, we learn how significant it is that we be capable of caring for one another through the office of medicine. For through our bodies we are forced to face our need for one another, and through learning to acknowledge that need we discover our "control" comes only through trust in others.

In summary, medicine is a practice embodying goods of health and care of the ill that gives those who have learned that practice rightful authority. Physicians have authority because they draw on the wisdom we have in common as bodily beings. Specialization, or, preferably, the calling of some members of the community to become physicians, is justified by the community's need to have some of its members committed to learning and practicing the skills of health and the means to care for the ill. That such a calling is required and justified indicates the kind of knowledge which can be gained through learning from the body, as well as the kind of skills necessary to care for individuals who are ill. This knowledge and these skills are not universal truths that can be known by just anyone. Rather, they are matters of learned judgments and wisdom which can only be sustained by those willing to place themselves under the guidance of an acknowledged master.

The Community of and Required by Medicine

Even if this account of medicine is persuasive (and there obviously are powerful challenges to the arguments raised here), it remains unclear whether these arguments successfully respond to MacIntyre's challenge. MacIntyre might even accept the construal of authority in medicine proposed in this essay but argue that what is lacking is a wider community and/or morality sufficient to sustain and support such a medicine. This response is apropos, but it is important to understand why.

As suggested earlier, physicians like Cassell insist that one of medicine's tasks is to teach us how to die. This task is drawn from the authority of the body. But in the absence of any consensus of what an appropriate death morally involves, how can any profession be entrusted with such an important task? It is no wonder that in the absence of such consensus or community the medical profession is tempted to become a self-protective interest group which tries to secure unwarranted power over our lives by claiming to be in possession of a knowledge peculiar to itself. It tries to justify its power by being what it cannot be—a science that frees us from, rather than teaches us, the limits of our bodies. This is not really the result of increasing technological power. Instead, increasing technological power is an attempt to maintain the moral coherence of medicine in a morally incoherent society—that is, medicine gains its moral coherence by drawing on the fear of death, the one thing people still seem to have in common. As a result, rather than a profession which provides assistance in living with the body, medicine becomes the modern analogue to the Gnostic heresy.[28]

Put differently, a medicine which assumes that its first task is to carry the wisdom of the body cannot help but challenge the assumptions that are at the heart of liberalism. This point can be illustrated by calling attention to the difficulty as well as necessity of physicians avowing their fallibility. That such an avowal is necessary is implied in the commitment to care for individual patients. This commitment involves contingent judgments which in principle exclude certainty.[29] Of course, some judgments can be more assured than others, but in principle physicians know they are making judgments for which they cannot claim infallibility.[30] Therefore, the physician's pledge to the patient (or perhaps more appropriately, the *covenant* that the physician and patient enter) does not include a guarantee of errorless judgment, but is rather a pledge of steadfast presence and care.

The avowal of fallibility by physicians is also necessitated through their commitment to learning how better to care for their patients, which is not the same thing as the growth of medical knowledge. Good patient care, as well as good science, depends on willingness to expose what does not work as readily as that which works. Failure is actually more important than success. Consequently, what is good for medicine as a profession may be disquieting to the patient who sees the physician as savior. Patients have to learn that they cannot assume that the care of physicians can be without error.[31] Indeed, patients must face the possibility that the best possible medicine of the day may be the wrong thing for them.[32] This is no reason to reject the care the physician can offer, but it does change decisively the attitude with which that care should be approved.

Yet as I have tried to suggest, in a society like ours which has no common account of goods, such a practice of medicine cannot be easily sustained. Medicine as a profession can only exist when it is also supported by a community that has a commitment to care even in the face of death. Such a community must not presuppose that the task of medicine is to keep illness and death at bay, as if such a task were an end in itself. Rather, the community should recognize that medicine involves those skills which allow its members to continue pursuing the goods of that community. Thus, a fallible medicine is sustained not only because this medicine serves the common good, but also because participation is a form of service for the whole community.

The absence of such a community in actuality, however, has meant that medicine (as MacIntyre suggests) increasingly has been forced to take the form of a contract between patient and physician. Contracts are the moral substitutes for modern society's lack of shared moral tradition. Of necessity medicine continues to insist that it is a self-sufficient institution, at least in part as an attempt to preserve its past commitment to the service of individual patients. As a result:

> it develops and maintains in the profession a self-deceiving view of the objectivity and reliability of its knowledge and the virtues of its members. Furthermore, it encourages the profession to see itself as the sole possessor of knowledge and virtue, to be somewhat suspicious of the technical and moral capacity of other occupations, and to be at best patronizing and at worst contemptuous of its clientele. Protecting the

profession from the demands of interaction on a free and equal basis with those in the world outside, its autonomy leads the profession to so distinguish its own virtue from those outside as to be unable to even perceive the need for, let alone undertake, the self-regulation it promises. ([8], p. 370)

Until now the only solution to this dilemma has been to demand more patient "autonomy," so that the patient can be protected from the physician and vice versa. This strategy is doomed to fail since the contract between physician and patient can never be "voluntary," in that the very condition which encourages patients to seek their physician's help is coercive. Physicians are also bound to this contract by the fact that, in their state of submission, patients expect the impossible. Once physicians fail, as they inevitably will, patients will blame them. The result can only be higher and higher malpractice insurance.

There seems to be little possibility of breaking this vicious cycle of false expectations and correlatively distorted forms of authority and power. At least for a while we will continue to be able to live off the capital of the past, but I suspect such a strategy cannot last much longer. MacIntyre suggests that one possible strategy would be to work with "those with whom one does share sufficient beliefs to rescue and to recreate authority within community that will break with the pluralist ethos. In medicine it means working for a variety of new forms of medical community, each with its own shared moral allegiance. With these the notion of authority could again begin to find context and content" ([12], p. 212).

This strategy might also have the unexpected effect of aiding in understanding the relationship between religious and medical communities. Ironically, the appropriate sense of the authority of medicine probably is not unrelated to the authority of the clergy mentioned at the beginning of this essay. The ability of a community to sustain a fallible medicine, a medicine that understands its first task to be mediating between us and our bodies—of carrying the wisdom of our finitude—is ultimately dependent on convictions about goods that set the task of medicine within a larger framework. When these goods are not seen to exist, or at least are ignored, medicine is tempted to become an end in itself. It thus becomes a pseudo-salvific institution.

In other words, medicine requires the existence of another institution to be able to keep its extremely significant, but limited, task *limited*. This does not mean that religious convictions should be supported in order to sustain medicine. Indeed, such functional justifications of religious beliefs are ill-advised. (If religious beliefs are false, then they should not be entertained no matter what good results they might engender.) Yet the fact that medicine as a practice requires convictions and institutions beyond itself to sustain its activity at least helps us understand why we are constantly tempted to ask too much of medicine in our secular times.

NOTES

1. Aspects of modern medicine correspond to each of Weber's types, but this should not be surprising since as "types" they are not meant to be mutually exclusive. For an analysis of medicine that draws more directly from Weber's theory of monopolization, see Berlant [2].

2. One of the difficulties with this topic involves how one should draw the distinction between authority *in* medicine and authority *of* medicine. Most of the current discussion is concerned with the latter, but the former is possibly more important. The question of authority in medicine seems to involve organizational and procedural questions internal to the profession, while authority of medicine concerns questions of the profession (and its representatives) over those who are recipients of medical care. Questions about the nature and legitimacy of each kind of authority are certainly different, but not unrelated. The authority *of* medicine depends for its legitimacy on claims about how authority functions *in* medicine. It becomes evident that part of the issue involving the authority of medicine is whether medicine ever has been the sort of practice capable of maintaining internal authority or whether, even if it once had the capability, it still is able to maintain it. Bosk [4] contends that the authority of attending physicians over their subordinates in surgery is not ultimately based on technical skill (though that must surely be present), but rather resides in their moral commitment:

> The professional's last line of defense is a moral one because it is a proper moral performance alone that substantiates a claim to proper technical performance when events mock such a claim. Moral error breaches a professional's contract with his client. He has not acted in good faith. He has done less than he should have. Such conduct is not honest and defensible but undercuts all the presumptions on which the professional-client relationship is based. For this reason moral errors are treated more seriously than technical ones. Hence the control of technical performance

is subordinated to the control of moral performance; without the over-arching moral system, the technical system is not amenable to control. ([4], p. 171)

Bosk's study as a whole is an impressive counter to the often-made claim that physicians receive almost no ethical training; he documents well that "post-graduate training of surgeons is above all things an ethical training" (p. 190). Thus, technical error can be forgiven, but not moral error.

3. See, for example, Nisbet [14] and Sennett [16]. One of the fasci-nating aspects of recent discussions of this topic is how similar the analysis of this social "problem" is from those on the political left and right.

4. ([3]), p. 67). Blum's book is meant to be a guide to help the doctor better "manage" the patient, but in fact it is an extremely useful account of the kinds of skills required if medicine is to be a legitimate practice. Thus, Blum argues that "the physician who fails to act as educator will be opening up the floodgates of disaster, both for himself and for his patient. Proper management of the relationship requires that the patient be an informed treatment partner of the doctor, one who knows what the basic assumptions of the profession and practice of medicine are, and one who knows something about the general content, and limits of knowledge about the human body" ([3], pp. 287-288). Of course Blum fails to note that such a patient might prove difficult to "manage."

5. Thus, Eliot Freidson maintains that "by virtue of being the author-ity on what illness 'really' is, medicine creates the social possibilities for act-ing sick. In this sense, medicine's monopoly includes the right to create ill-ness as an official social role. It is part of being a profession to be given the official power to define and therefore create the shape of problematic segments of social behavior" ([8], p. 206). Freidson is not denying that disease involves biophysical processes, but is pointing out that when it is defined as an illness by medicine it is changed: "Thus, when a veterinarian diagnoses a cow's con-dition as an illness, he does not merely by diagnosis change the cow's behavior: to the cow, illness remains as an experienced biophysical state; no more. But when a physician diagnoses a human's condition as illness, he changes the man's behavior by diagnosis: a social state is added to a biophysical state by assigning the meaning of illness to disease" ([8], p. 223).

6. See, for example, Berlant's compelling analysis of the development of medical ethics from Percival's code to the present day as a study of the legitimation of medical monopolization ([2], pp. 64–127).

7. For a good example of the political implications of this supposition, see Dahl [7]. What proponents of such a view often fail to realize is that autonomy itself is a form of authority which can be as destructive as pater-nalism. For a sensitive discussion of autonomy as a form of authority, see

Sennett ([16], pp. 84–121). Sennett suggests that the stress on autonomy forces all human relationships to be understood as forms of manipulation to maintain dominance. He states that

> when a person is needed by others more than he needs them, he can afford to be indifferent to them. If the bureaucrat ignores the distress of the welfare client filling out complicated forms, if the doctor treats his clients like bodies rather than persons, these very acts of indifference maintain dominance. In the complex form of autonomy, keeping cool when others make demands on you or challenge you is a way of keeping the upper hand. Of course, few people set out to be rude or callous. But autonomy removes the necessity of dealing with other people openly and mutually. There is an imbalance, they show their need for you more than you show your need for them. This puts you in control. ([16], p. 86).

Sennett thus argues that appeals to autonomy as a way to legitimize certain relations is an illusion, because such appeals disguise the fact that one side holds more power. This imbalance often goes unnoticed, though, because it is assumed that in an autonomous relationship there is no power present—or if present, it is legitimate since it is exercised "impersonally" ([16], pp. 104–116).

8. I certainly do not intend my argument to be an apology for everything done in the name of modern medicine. If applied consistently, the position developed in this essay would require some profound changes in the practice and institutionalization of medicine. However, I have tried to present my argument in a positive manner, since what we need is not another diatribe about what is wrong with medicine, but some sense of what constuctively needs to be done.

9. MacIntyre suggests that this understanding of scientific authority is very similar to some accounts of church authority—particularly in relation to doctrinal development. I suspect he is right and that the analysis of the similarities and differences would prove to be an extremely fruitful enterprise. For an attempt to understand the authority of scripture in a similar manner, see Hauerwas ([9], pp. 53–71). The analogy of science and theological development may not be entirely happy, however, as it tends to suggest that tradition always grows in a positive direction. That is by no means the case. In fact, one of the remarkable things about Scripture is the inclusion in the text itself of the mistaken directions tradition has taken. Even more importantly, Scripture does not make clear in itself which were the mistakes and which were the successes. Thus it is necessary for each new generation to struggle with and continue the arguments begun in Scripture itself.

10. I simply do not have the competence to state, much less defend,

the epistemological assumptions underlying this claim. I assume, with Aristotle, that ethics deals with "matters that can be other," and that it does so is not an epistemological liability, except for those who assume that necessary knowledge is paradigmatic of truth. Moreover, I assume that much of our knowledge, such as that in medicine, is more like moral knowledge than certain epistemological theories assume. However, this does not mean that such knowledge is in any way deficient or false.

11. ([12], pp. 199–200). Bosk points out that there are "two competing systems of legitimation for medical authority: clinical expertise and scientific evidence. These systems are not of equal importance: in the case of discrepant opinion, arguments based on clinical expertise override those based on scientific evidence." That is why medical training inherently requires apprenticeship to a master, since it is only through the master that one can acquire the experience necessary for the training of judgment.

12. MacIntyre defines a practice as "any coherent and complex form of socially established cooperative human activity through which goods internal to that form of activity are realized in the course of trying to achieve those standards of excellence which are appropriate to, and partially definitive of, that form of activity, with the result that human powers to achieve excellence, and human conceptions of the ends and goods involved, are systematically extended. Tic-tac-toe is not an example of a practice in this sense, nor is throwing a football with skill; but the game of football is, and so is chess. Planting turnips is not a practice; farming is" ([11], p. 175).

Practices have standards, of course, though they are not immune from criticism. It is still true, however, that we cannot be initiated into a practice without accepting the authority of the best standards to date for that practice. That is why it is essential to note that practices have a history, as they are not constituted by goals fixed for all time, but the goals themselves are transmuted by the history of practice. MacIntyre's analysis of practice is crucial for his understanding of virtue, since the latter is "an acquired human quality the possession and exercise of which tends to enable us to achieve those goods which are internal to practices and the lack of which effectively prevents us from achieving any such goods" ([11], p. 178).

13. MacIntyre clearly identifies medicine as a practice, and I think he is correct to do so.

14. See also Simon ([18], pp. 144–194).

15. Dahl ([7], p. 8). It is very interesting to note that Dahl's example of the "criteria of competence" as a qualification of the "criteria of choice" is that of medicine.

16. There are further issues involved in MacIntyre's view that can only be mentioned in this context: the question of the relation of a practice to an institution and the problem of the unity or possible conflict between the

virtues. In terms of the first question, MacIntyre maintains that practices must not be confused with institutions, since the latter are characteristically concerned with external goods. No practice can survive without institutions, as they characteristically form a single causal order; yet, that such is the case means a practice is constantly open to distortion. That is why the virtues are essential, since without them a practice cannot resist the corrupting power of institutions ([11], p. 181). Against Plato, MacIntyre maintains the possibility of the conflict of virtues. That is why our "situation is tragic in that we have to recognize the authority of both claims. There is an objective moral order, but our perceptions of it are such that we cannot bring rival moral truths into complete harmony" ([11], p. 134). That is why we require a community capable of maintaining the necessary conversation between practices, each of which we may need, but which are in potential if not actual conflict. Moreover, the very need for specialization assumes added importance from this perspective, because often the specializations reflect different virtues which society needs, but which may be in conflict. Accordingly, a morally healthy society may well be one that is able to sustain the necessary tension between professions.

   17. ([12], p. 207). I am not denying, of course, that physicians' expertise is relevant to their authority. Rather, I am suggesting that this expertise is relevant only within a more determinative moral framework.

   18. However, Blum documents that most patients attribute authority to physicians today primarily because they are considered such "experts" ([3], pp. 81 ff.). That is part of the reason attempts to define a "profession" are so inconclusive. A profession is inherently a normative concept denoting service to the basic goods which a particular community thinks are essential for its moral identity. The reason many specializations which require perhaps even more skill than the traditional professions still are not professions is that they are not essential to the community's moral purpose — though they may be to its physical survival.

   19. For a more extended analysis of this point, see Hauerwas ([9], pp. 111–127). I cannot pretend, however, to have dealt sufficiently with all the issues raised by suggesting that a relation is capable of being qualified by a virtue.

   20. See, for example, Eric Cassell's claims in this respect ([6], pp. 87, 113). Of course, I am not denying that various illnesses involve normative judgment, but I am suggesting the idea of "health" as a clear and distinct idea is a chimera. At the same time, however, I think those who construe all characterizations of illness as arbitrary cannot be right. No doubt "illness" is often a culturally relative designation but a broken arm is still a broken arm.

   21. From this perspective one of the most overlooked aspects of our current situation is how medical schools continue to function as schools of

virtue. They are among the few institutions in our society that have a coherent enough purpose that enables them to form character. I only wish we could exhibit the same kind of self-confidence in our seminaries.

22. This fact may be one of the reasons that medicine and religion are always interrelated. Each deals with the same subject, but in different ways. Both are tempted to deny the special task of the other in hopes of being the sole authority. In truth, neither can be helpful without the other.

23. For a particularly compelling account of the notion of "embodiment" and its implications for medicine, see Richard Zaner ([20]. Zaner's analysis is particularly helpful in suggesting how a body is at once "mine" and yet "not mine," but nonetheless not an object that can be placed over or against a person.

24. Again the church provides a useful illustration in this respect. The more specialized the function of the clergy became from that of the laity, the more the potential for the illegitimation of the priesthood itself. The more laity viewed their clergy's roles as foreign to their own lives, the more likely it became that the roles of the priests would be associated with magic and/or arbitrary power. This would result finally in either rejection or legitimacy, the latter by making Christianity a mystery cult. With rejection laity are no better off, because too often clerical authority is rejected in the name of an equally destructive authority which offers a bogus salvation. The technological form of contemporary medicine involves many of the same dangers. The more laity are prevented from understanding what is being done to them in the name of science, the more likely they are to turn to alternative forms of care. Quackery and purely technological medicine are but two sides of the same coin. From the laity's perspective they are judged by the same criterion — results.

25. Cassell's examples are not just illustrations — they are the argument, and rightly so. Contrary to the most contemporary accounts of argument, I assume that good arguments cannot be separated from the context that makes them intelligible in the first place. It would take me too far afield to develop this point, but stated briefly it involves the contention that there exists no foundational point on which arguments as such rest. Rather, all arguments begin in the midst of things and are proved true or false exactly by how plausibly they display the narratives on which they depend. For a more thorough defense of this view, see David Burrell [5].

26. No doubt Cassell means that when people are faced with illness or death they exhibit what they want and what they are. But I think it wrong to suggest this is a challenge to social convention, since what we really want and are is itself a convention. Conventions are sometimes lies, but they are also just as likely to be the way to truth.

27. Cassell's way of putting this is an interesting case of someone's in-

sight fighting against its own expression. Although Cassell uses the word *soar*, the very examples he uses (polio victims' struggles to retain some control over their bodies) suggest that "soaring" is really more a matter of learning to live at peace with the body. The same kind of problem occurs in Cassell's defense of the importance of the "omnipotence" of physicians for helping patients recover their own omnipotence. Yet Cassell's own critique of the dangers of such omnipotence for physician and patient alike suggests that the control patients seek is not so much omnipotence as simply the power to make their lives their own ([6], pp. 142–145).

28. Gnosticism was not only a Christian heresy, but a widespread and extremely complex phenomenon in the ancient world. No simple generalization can be sufficient to characterize Gnostic beliefs or practices. By suggesting that some aspects of modern medicine bear close analogy to Gnosticism I mean no more than: (1) medicine, like Gnosticism, is often seen, at least implicitly, as offering a form of salvation; (2) that such salvation is obtained through esoteric knowledge possessed by those who have a special training; and (3) that the salvation offered is basically an attempt to free us from the limits of our bodies.

29. ([15], p. 124). Actually, Bosk [4] presents the most complete analysis of error in medicine. He distinguishes between *technical errors*, which are expected to happen to everyone and which must thus be quickly reported; *judgmental errors*, which involve clinical judgments; and *normative* and *quasi-normative errors*, which involve a failure to fulfill the moral expectations of the physician's role. In medicine *technical error* must be exposed and forgiven, since only in that way can the failure be prevented from happening again ([4], p. 128). Thus Bosk notes that "Grand Rounds" and "Mortality and Morbidity Conferences" are actually elaborate rituals "the entire congregation of surgeons have evolved for witnessing them [errors], resolving the confusion they create, and incorporating them into the group's history and the individual's biography" ([4], p. 121).

30. Pellegrino's and Thomasma's account of clinical judgments is particularly worth reading, as is their argument for the necessity of discretionary space in professional judgments ([15], pp. 155–169). For a particularly biting critique of the model of the clinician as requiring personal judgment to justify the "autonomy" of the physician, see Freidson ([8], pp. 346–349). However, Bosk's study of how medical students are trained to assume the moral role of "professional self-control" at least qualifies Freidson's critique. Bosk points out, "The problem is not, as some have claimed, an absence of any socialization, controls, or ethical sense in the profession; the problem is rather a system which celebrates individual conscience as a control while ignoring corporate responsibility. The profession of medicine needs to develop structural remedies — or structure socialization — in a way that brings into balance both

the corporate and the individual dimensions of control" ([4], p. 188).

31. I have not discussed the implications of my analysis of the authority of medicine for the specification of and/or relation between the various roles in medicine—e.g., physician, nurse, counselor. I think no *a priori* formula exists by which this can be done. Different roles develop historically as part of medicine's conversation with itself or are governed by changing needs of patients. However, the current dominance of the physician—in part justified by their technical expertise—or the attempt of the physician to usurp all other roles is dangerous for the physician as well as the patient. If the physician is "first among equals," he is so because of the need to have someone morally responsible, not simply because of his expertise.

32. It is interesting that Bosk only treats the necessity of surgeons to expose errors among themselves. He does not ask if error should also be exposed to the patient and, if so, what would be the implications of such exposure.

REFERENCES

[1] Beauchamp, T., and Childress, J. 1979. *Principles of Biomedical Ethics.* New York and Oxford: Oxford University Press.

[2] Berlant, J. L. 1975. *Profession and Monopoly.* Berkeley: University of California Press.

[3] Blum, R. 1960. *The Management of the Doctor-Patient Relationship.* New York: McGraw-Hill.

[4] Bosk, C. L. 1979. *Forgive and Remember: Managing Medical Failure.* Chicago: University Press.

[5] Burrell, D. 1981. "Argument in Theology: Analogy and Narrative." In Carl Rashchke, ed., *New Dimensions in Philosophy of Religion*, (37-52). Chico, Ca.: Scholars Press.

[6] Cassell, E. 1976. *The Healer's Art: A New Approach to the Doctor-Patient Relationship.* Philadelphia: Lippincott.

[7] Dahl, R. 1970. *After the Revolution?* New Haven: Yale University Press.

[8] Freidson, E. 1970. *Profession of Medicine.* New York: Harper and Row.

[9] Hauerwas, S. 1981. *A Community of Character.* Notre Dame, Ind.: University of Notre Dame Press.

[10] Hauerwas, S. 1978. "Religious Concepts of Brain Death and Associated Problems," *New York Academy of Sciences Annals* 215: 329–338. Reprinted in the present volume (see essay no. 4)

[11] MacIntyre, A. 1981. *After Virtue: A Study in Moral Theory.* Notre Dame, Ind.: University of Notre Dame Press.

[12] MacIntyre, A. 1977. "Patients as Agents." In H. T. Engelhardt, Jr., and S.F. Spicker, eds., *Philosophical Medical Ethics: Its Nature and the Significance*, 197-212. Dordrecht, Holland: Reidel.

[13] May, W. 1977. "Code and Covenant or Philanthropy and Contract?" In W. Curran, A. Dyke, S. Reiser, eds., *Ethics in Medicine: Historical Perspectives and Contemporary Concerns*, 65-76. Cambridge, Mass.: MIT Press.
[14] Nisbet, R. 1975. *Twilight of Authority*. New York: Oxford University Press.
[15] Pellegrino, E. D., and Thomasma, D.C. 1981. *A Philosophical Basis of Medical Practice*. New York: Oxford University Press.
[16] Sennett, R. 1980. *Authority*. New York: Alfred Knopf.
[17] Simon, Y. 1980. *A General Theory of Authority*. Notre Dame, Ind.: University of Notre Dame Press.
[18] Simon, Y. 1951. *Philosophy of Democratic Government*. Chicago: University of Chicago Press.
[19] Weber, Max. 1958. "The Social Psychology of the World Religions." In H. H. Gerth and C. W. Mills, eds., *Max Weber: Essays in Sociology*, 295-301. New York: Oxford University Press.
[20] Zaner, R. 1978. "Embodiment." In W. Reich, ed., *Encyclopedia of Bioethics*, 361-365. New York: Free Press.

3

Salvation and Health:
Why Medicine Needs the Church

A Text and a Story

While it is not unheard of for a theologian to begin an essay with a text from the Scripture, it is relatively rare for those who are addressing issues of medicine to do so. However I begin with a text, as almost everything I have to say is but a commentary on this passage from Job 2:11–13:

> Now when Job's friends heard of all this evil that had come upon him, then came each from his own place, Eliphaz the Temanite, Bildad the Shuhite, and Zophar the Na'amathite. They made an appointment together to come console with him and comfort him. And when they saw him from afar, they did not recognize him; and they raised their voices and wept; and they rent their robes and sprinkled dust upon their heads toward heaven. And they sat with him on the ground seven days and seven nights, and no one spoke a word to him, for they saw that his suffering was very great.

I do not want to comment immediately on the text. Instead, I think it best to begin by telling you a story. The story is about one of my earliest friendships. When I was in my early teens I had a friend, let's call him Bob, who meant everything to me. We made our first hesitant steps toward growing up through sharing the things young boys do—i.e., double dating, athletic activities, and endless discussions on every topic. For two years we were inseparable. I was extremely appreciative of Bob's friendship, as he was not only brighter and more talented than I, but also came from a family that was economically considerably better off than my own. Through Bob I was introduced to a world that otherwise I would hardly know existed. For example, we spent hours in his home playing pool in a room that was built for no other purpose; and we swam in the lake that his house was specifically built to overlook.

Then very early one Sunday morning I received a phone call from Bob requesting that I come to see him immediately. He was sobbing intensely but through his crying he was able to tell me that they had just found his mother dead. She had committed suicide by placing a shotgun in her mouth. I knew immediately I did not want to go to see him and/or confront a reality like that. I had not yet learned the desperation hidden under our everyday routines and I did not want to learn of it. Moreover I did not want to go because I knew there was nothing I could do or say to make things even appear better than they were. Finally I did not want to go because I did not want to be close to anyone who had been touched by such a tragedy.

But I went. I felt awkward, but I went. And as I came into Bob's room we embraced, a gesture that was almost unheard of between young men raised in the Southwest, and we cried together. After that first period of shared sorrow we somehow calmed down and took a walk. For the rest of that day and that night we stayed together. I do not remember what we said, but I do remember that it was inconsequential. We never talked about his mother or what had happened. We never speculated about why she might do such a thing, even though I could not believe someone who seemed to have such a good life would want to die. We did what we always did. We talked girls, football, cars, movies, and anything else that was inconsequential enough to distract our attention from this horrible event.

As I look on that time I now realize that it was obviously one of the most important events in my life. That it was so is at least partly indicated by how often I have thought about it and tried to under- stand its significance in the years from then to now. As often as I have reflected on what happened in that short space of time I have also remembered how inept I was in helping Bob. I did not know what should or could be said. I did not know how to help him start sorting out such a horrible event so that he could go on. All I could do was be present.

But time has helped me realize that this is all he wanted—namely, my presence. For as inept as I was, my willingness to be present was a sign that this was not an event so horrible that it drew us away from all other human contact. Life could go on, and in the days to follow we would again swim together, double date, and generally waste time. I now think that at the time God granted me the marvelous privilege of being a presence in the face of profound pain and suffering even when I did not appreciate the significance of being present.

Yet the story cannot end here. For while it is true that Bob and I did go on being friends, nothing was the same. For a few months we continued to see one another often, but somehow the innocent joy of loving one another was gone. We slowly found that our lives were going in different directions and we developed new friends. No doubt the difference between our social and cultural opportunities helps explain to some extent our drifting apart. Bob finally went to Princeton and I went to Southwestern University in Georgetown, Texas.

But that kind of explanation for our growing apart is not sufficient. What was standing between us was that day and night we spent together under the burden of a profound sadness that neither of us had known could exist until that time. We had shared a pain so intense that for a short period we had become closer than we knew, but now the very pain that created that sharing stood in the way of the development of our friendship. Neither of us wished to recapture that time, nor did we know how to make that night and day part of our ongoing story together. So we went our separate ways. I have no idea what became of Bob, though every once in a while I remember to ask my mother if she has heard about him.

Does medicine need the church? How could this text and this story possibly help us understand that question, much less suggest how it might be answered? Yet I am going to claim in this essay that it does. Put briefly, what I will try to show is that if medicine can be rightly understood as an activity that trains some to know how to be present to those in pain, then something very much like a church is needed to sustain that presence day in and day out. Before I try to develop that thesis, however, I need to do some conceptual groundbreaking to make clear exactly what kind of claim I am trying to make about the relationship of salvation and health, medicine and the church.

Religion and Medicine: Is There or Should There Be a Relation?

It is a well-known fact that for most of human history there has been a close affinity between religion and medicine. Indeed that very way of putting it is misleading, since to claim a relation suggests that they were distinguished, and often that has not been the case. From earliest times, disease and illness were not seen as matters having no religious import but rather as resulting from the disfavor of God. As Darrel Amundsen and Gary Ferngren have recently reminded us, the Hebrew Scriptures often depict God promising

> health and prosperity for the covenant people if they are faithful to him, and disease and other suffering if they spurn his love. This promise runs through the Old Testament. "If you will diligently hearken to the voice of the Lord your God, and do that which is right in his eyes, and give heed to his commandments and keep all his statutes, I will put none of the diseases upon you which I put upon the Egyptians; for I am the Lord, your healer" (Exod. 15:26). ([2], p. 92)

This view of illness was not associated only with the community as a whole, but with individuals. Thus in Psalm 38 the lament is

> There is no soundness in my flesh because of thy indignation; there is no health in my bones because of my sin. . . . My wounds grow foul and fester because of foolishness. . . . I am utterly spent and crushed; I groan because of the tumult of my heart. . . . Do not forsake me, O Lord! O my God, be not far from me! Make haste to help me, O Lord, my salvation! (vv. 3, 5, 8, 21–22)

Amundsen and Ferngren point out this view of illness as accompanied by the assumption that acknowledgment of and repentence for our sin was essential for our healing. Thus in Psalm 32:

> When I declared not my sin, my body wasted away through my groaning all day long. For day and night thy hand was heavy upon me; my strength was dried up. . . . I acknowledged my sin to thee, and I did not hide my iniquity; I said, "I will confess my transgressions to the Lord"; then thou didst forgive the guilt of my sin. (vv. 3–5) ([2], p. 93)

Since illness and sin were closely connected it is not surprising that healing was also closely associated with religious practices—or, put more accurately, healing was a religious discipline. Indeed Amundsen and Ferngren make the interesting point that since the most important issue was a person's relationship with God the chief means of healing was naturally prayer. That clearly precluded magic and thus the Mosaic code excluded soothsayers, augurs, sorcerers, charmers, wizards, and other such figures who offered a means to control or avoid the primary issue of their relation to Yahweh ([2], p. 94). They also suggest that this may have been why no sacerdotal medical practice developed in Israel particularly associated with the priesthood. Rather, the pattern of the Exodus tended to prevail, with illness and healing more closely associated with prophetic activity.

The early Christian community seems to have done little to change these basic presuppositions. If anything it simply intensified them by adding what Amundsen and Ferngren call the "central paradox" in the New Testament:

> Strength comes only through weakness. This strength is Christ's strength that comes only through dependence upon him. In the Gospel of John, Christ says: "I have said to you, that in me you may have peace. In the world you have tribulation; but be of good cheer, I have overcome the world" (16:33). "In the world you have tribulation." It is simply to be expected and accepted. But for the New Testament Christian no suffering is meaningless. The ultimate purpose and meaning behind Christian suffering in the New Testament is spiritual maturity. And the ultimate goal in spiritual maturity is a close dependence upon Christ based upon a childlike trust. ([2], p. 96)

Thus illness is seen as an opportunity for growth in faith and trust in God.

Because of this way of viewing both the positive and negative effect of illness, Amundsen and Ferngren note that there has always been a degree of tension in the way Christians understand the relation between theology and secular medicine, between the medicine of the soul and the medicine of the body.

> According to one view, if God sends disease either to punish or to test a person, it is to God that one must turn for care and healing. If God is both the source and healer of a person's ills, the use of human medicine would circumvent the spiritual framework by resorting to worldly wisdom. On another view, if God is the source of disease, or if God permits disease and is the ultimate healer, God's will can be fulfilled through human agents, who with divine help have acquired the ability to aid in the curative process. Most Christians have asserted that the human agent of care, the physician, is an instrument of God, used by God in bringing succor to humankind. But in every age some have maintained that any use of human medicine is a manifestation

of a lack of faith. This ambivalence in the Christian attitude, among both theologians and laity, has always been present to some degree. ([2], p. 96)

Nor is it possible to separate or distinguish religion and medicine on the basis of a distinction between soul and body. For as Paul Ramsey has reminded us, Christians affirm that God has created and holds us sacred as embodied souls ([14], p. xiii). Religion does not deal with the soul and medicine with the body. Practitioners of both are too well aware of the inseparability of soul and body—or perhaps better, they know the abstractness of both categories. Moreover when religion too easily legitimates the independence of medical care by limiting medicine to mechanical understanding and care of the body, it has the result of making religious convictions ethereal in character. It may be that just to the extent Christianity is always tempted in Gnostic and Manichean directions it accepts too willingly a technological understanding of medicine. Christians, if they are to be faithful to their convictions, may not ever be able to avoid at least potential conflict between their own assumptions about illness and health and how the ill should be cared for and the assumptions of medicine. One hopes for cooperation, of course, but structurally the possibility of conflict between church and medicine cannot be excluded, since both entail convictions and practices concerned with that same subject.

Put differently, given Judaism and Christianity's understanding of humankind's relation with God—that is: how we understand salvation—health can never be thought of as an autonomous sphere. Moreover, insofar as medicine is a specialized activity distinguished from religious convictions, you cannot exclude the possibility that there may well be conflict between religion and medicine. For in many ways the latter is constantly tempted to offer a form of salvation that religiously may come close to idolatry. The ability of modern medicine to cure is at once a benefit and potential pitfall. Too often it is tempted to increase its power by offering more than care, by offering in fact alleviation from the human condition—e.g., the development of artificial hearts. That is not the fault of medical practitioners, though often they encourage such idolatry; rather the fault lies with those of us who pretentiously place undue expectations on medicine in the hope of finding an earthly remedy to our death. But we can never forget that the relation between medicine and health, and especially the health of a population, is as ambiguous as the relation between the church and salvation.

In the hope of securing peace between medicine and religion, two quite different and equally unsatisfactory proposals have been suggested. The first advocates a strong division of labor between medicine and religion by limiting the scope of medicine to the mechanism of our body. While it is certainly true that medicine in a unique way entails the passing on of the wisdom of the body from one generation to another, there is no way that medical care can be limited to the body and be good medicine [10]. As Ramsey has reminded us again and again, the moral commitment of the physician is not to treat diseases, or populations, or the human race, but the immediate patient before him or her ([14], pp. 36, 59). Religiously, therefore, the care offered by physicians cannot be abstracted from the moral commitment to care based on our view that every aspect of our existence is dependent upon God.

By the same token the clergy, no less than physicians, are concerned about the patient's physical well-being. No assumptions about technical skills and knowledge can legitimate the clergy retreating into the realm of the spiritual in order to claim some continued usefulness and status. Such a retreat is as unfaithful as abandoning the natural world to the physicist on the grounds that God is a God of history and not of nature. For the church and its officeholders to abandon claims over the body in the name of a lack of expertise is equivalent to reducing God to the gaps in scientific theory. Such a strategy is not only bad faith but it results in making religious convictions appear at best irrelevant and at worse foolish.

The second alternative to accepting the autonomy of medicine from our religious convictions seeks to maintain a close relationship by resacralizing medical care. Medicine requires a "holistic vision of man" ([7], p. 9), because the care it brings is but one aspect of salvation. Thus the church and its theology serves medical care by promoting a holistic view of man, one that can provide a

> comprehensive understanding of human health [that] includes the greatest possible harmony of all of man's forces and energies, the greatest possible spiritualization of man's bodily aspect and the finest embodi-

ment of the spiritual. True health is revealed in the self-actualization
of the person who has attained that freedom which marshals all available
energies for the fulfillment of his total human vocation. ([7], p. 154)

Such a view of health, however, cannot help but pervert the kind
of care that physicians can provide. Physicians rightly maintain that
their skill primarily has to do with the body, as medicine promises
us health, not happiness. When such a general understanding of health
is made the goal of medicine, it only results in making medical care
promise more than it can deliver. As a result, we are tyrannized by
the agents of medicine because we have voluntarily vested them with
too much power. It is already a difficult task in our society to control
the expectations people have about modern medicine; we only com-
pound that problem by providing religious legitimacy to this overblown
understanding of health. Certainly we believe that any account of salvation includes questions of our health, but that does not mean that
medicine can or ever should become the agency of salvation. It may
be a fundamental judgment on the church's failure to help us locate
wherein our salvation lies that so many today seek a salvation through
medicine.

Can Medical Ethics Be Christian?

The already complex question of the relation between religion
and medicine only becomes more confusing when we turn our attention to more recent developments in medical ethics. For even though
religious thinkers have been at the forefront of much of the work done
in the expanding field of "medical ethics," it is not clear that they
have been there as religious thinkers. Joseph Fletcher [5], Paul Ramsey
[14], James Gustafson [6], Charles Curran [4], Jim Childress [3], to
name just a few, have done extensive work in medical ethics, but often
it is hard to tell how their religious convictions have made a difference
for the methodology they employ or for their response to specific quandaries. Indeed it is interesting to note how seldom they raise issues
of the meaning or relation of salvation and health, as they seem to
prefer dealing with questions of death and dying, truth telling, etc.

By calling attention to this fact by no means do I wish to disparage
the kind of reflection that has been done concerning these issues. We
have all benefited from their careful analysis and distinctions concern-

ing such problems. Yet one must wonder if, by letting the agenda be set in such a manner, we have already lost the theological ball game. For the very concentration on "issues" and "quandaries" as central for medical ethics tends to underwrite the practice of medicine as we know it, rather than challenging some of the basic presuppositions of medical practice and care. Because of this failure to raise more fundamental questions, concerns that might provide more access for our theological claims are simply never considered.

There are at least two reasons for this that I think are worth mentioning. The first has to do with the character of theological ethics itself. We tend to forget that the development of "Christian ethics" is a relatively new development [8]. It has only been in the last hundred years that some have styled themselves as "ethicists" rather than simply theologians. It is by no means clear that we know how to indicate what difference it makes conceptually and methodologically to claim our ethics as Christian in distinction from other kinds of ethical reflection. In the hopes of securing greater clarity about their own work many who have identified their work as Christian have nonetheless assumed that the meaning and method of "ethics" was determined fundamentally by non-Christian sources. In a sense the very concentration on "medical ethics" was a godsend for many "religious ethicists," as it seemed to provide a coherent activity without having to deal with the fundamental issue of what makes Christian ethics Christian.

This can be illustrated by attending to the debate among Christian ethicists concerning whether Christian moral reasoning is primarily deontological or consequential. This debate has been particularly important for medical ethics, as obviously how you think about non-therapeutic experimentation, truth-telling, transplants, and a host of other issues seems to turn on this issue. For instance, Joseph Fletcher, who wrote one of the first books by a Protestant in medical ethics, has always argued in favor of a consequential stance, thus qualifying the physician's commitment to an individual patient in the name of a greater good [5]. In contrast, Paul Ramsey has emphasized that the "covenant" of the physician with the patient is such that no amount of good to be done should override that commitment [14].

It is interesting to note how each makes theological appeals to support his own position. Fletcher appeals to love as his basic norm, interpreting it in terms of the greatest good for the greatest number, but it remains unclear how his sense of love is theologically warranted

or controlled. Ramsey provides a stronger theological case for his emphasis on "covenant" as a central theological motif, but it is not clear
how the many "covenants of life with life into which we are born"
require the covenant of God with a particular people we find in Scripture. Ramsey's use of covenant language thus underwrites a natural
law ethic whose status is unclear both from a theological and/or
philosophical perspective.[1]

What is interesting about the debate between Fletcher and Ramsey
is that it could have been carried on completely separate from the
theological premises that each side claimed were involved. For the terms
of the debate—*consequential* and *deontological*—are basically borrowed
from philosophical contexts and are dependent on the presuppositions
of certain philosophical traditions. Of course that in itself does not
mean that such issues and concepts are irrelevant to our work as theologians, but what is missing is any sense of how the issue as presented
grows, is dependent on, or informed by our distinctive commitments
as theologians.

The question of the nature of theological ethics and its relation
to the development of ethical reflection in and about medicine is further complicated by our current cultural situation. As Ramsey has
pointed out, we are currently trying to do the impossible—namely,
"build a civilization without an agreed civil tradition and [in] the
absence of a moral consensus" ([13], p. 15). This makes the practice
of medicine even more morally challenging, since it is by no means
clear how one can sustain a non-arbitrary medicine in a genuinely
morally pluralistic society. For example, much of the debate about when
someone is "really" dead is not simply the result of our increased
technological power to keep blood flowing through our bodies, but
witnesses to our culture's lack of consensus as to what constitutes a well-
lived life and the correlative sense of a good death. In the absence
of such a consensus our only recourse is to resort to claims and counter-
claims about "right to life" and "right to die," with the result of the
further impoverishment of our moral language and vision. Moreover,
the only way to create a "safe" medicine under such conditions is to
expect physicians to treat us as if death is the ultimate enemy to be
put off by every means. Then we blame physicians for keeping us alive
beyond all reason, but fail to note that if they did not we would not
know how to distinguish them from murderers.

Alasdair MacIntyre has raised this sort of issue directly in his "Can

Medicine Dispense with a Theological Perspective on Human Nature?" Rather than calling attention to what has become problematic for physicians and surgeons—issues such as when it is appropriate to let someone die—he says he wants to direct our attention to what is still taken for granted, "namely, the unconditional and absolute character of certain of the doctor's obligations to his patients" ([12], p. 120). The difficulty is that modern philosophy, according to MacIntyre, has been unable to offer a persuasive account of such an obligation.

> *Either* they distort and misrepresent it *or* they render it unintelligible. Teleological moralists characteristically end up by distorting and misrepresenting. For they begin with a notion of moral rules as specifying how we are to behave if we are to achieve certain ends, perhaps *the* end for man, the *summmum bonum*. If I break such rules I shall fail to achieve some human good and will thereby be frustrated and impoverished. ([12], p. 122)

But MacIntyre notes that this treats moral failure as if it is an educational failure and lacks the profound guilt that should accompany moral failure. More importantly, such an account fails entirely to account for the positive evil we know certain people clearly pursue.

Moral philosophers who tend to preserve the unconditional and absolute character of the central requirements of morality, however, inevitably make those "oughts" appear as if they are arbitrary. What they cannot do is show how those oughts are rationally entailed by an account of man's true end. Kant was only able to do so because he continued the presupposition (which he failed to justify within his own philosophical position) that "the life of the individual and also of that of the human race is a journey toward a goal" ([12], p. 127). Once that presupposition is lost, however, and MacIntyre believes that it has been lost in our culture, then we lack the resources to maintain exactly those moral presuppositions that seem essential to securing the moral integrity of medicine.

Such a situation seems ripe for a theological response, since it might at least be suggested that it thus becomes our task as theologians to serve our culture in general and medicine in particular by supplying the needed rationale. Yet, MacIntyre argues, such a strategy is doomed, since the very intelligibility of theological claims has been rendered problematic by the ethos of modernity. Therefore, just to the extent theologians try to make their claims in terms offered by modernity, they only underwrite the assumption that theological language cannot be meaningful.

This kind of dilemma is particularly acute when it comes to medicine. For if the theologian attempts to underwrite the medical ethos drawing on the particular convictions of Christians, just to the extent those convictions are particular they will serve only to emphasize society's lack of a common morality. Thus theologians, in the interest of cultural consensus, often try to downplay the distinctiveness of their theological convictions in the interest of societal harmony. But in the process we only reinforce the assumption on the part of many that theological claims make little difference for how medicine itself is understood or how various issues are approached. At best theology or religion is left with justifying a concern with the "whole patient," but it is not even clear how that concern depends on or derives from any substantive theological conviction that is distinguishable from humanism.

Almost as if we have sensed that there is no way to resolve this dilemma, theologians and religious professionals involved in medicine have tended to associate with the patients' rights movement. At least one of the ways of resolving our cultural dilemma is to protect the patient from medicine by restoring the patient's autonomy over against the physician. While I certainly do not want to underestimate the importance of patients recovering a sense of medicine as an activity in which we play as important a role as the physician, the emphasis on the patient's rights over against the physician cannot resolve our difficulty. It is but an attempt to substitute procedural safeguards for what only substantive convictions can supply. As a result our attention is distracted from the genuine challenge we confront for the forming of an ethos sufficient to sustain a practice of medicine that is morally worthy.

Pain, Loneliness, and Being Present: The Church and the Care of the Ill

I can offer no "solution" to the issues raised in the previous section, as I think they admit of no solution, given our social and political situation. Moreover, I think we will make little headway on such matters as long as we try to address the questions in terms of the dichotomies of religion and medicine or the relation between medical ethics and theology. Rather, what is needed is a restatement of the issue. In this section I will try to do that by returning to my original text and story to suggest how they may help remind us that more fundamental than questions of religion and morality is the question of the kind of community necessary to sustain the long-term care of the ill.

Indeed, part of the problem with discussing the question of "relation" in such general terms as "medicine" and "religion" is that each of those terms in its own way distorts the character of what it is meant to describe. For example, when we talk in general about "religion" rather than a specific set of beliefs, behaviors, and habits embodied by a distinct group of people, our account always tends to be reductionistic. It makes it appear that underlying what people actually believe and do is a deeper reality called "religion." It is as if we can talk about God abstracted from how a people have learned to pray to that God. In like manner we often tend to oversimplify the nature of medicine by trying to capture the many activities covered by that term in a definition or ideological system. What doctors do is often quite different from what they say they do.

Moreover, the question of the relation of theology to medical ethics is far too abstract. For when the issue is posed in that manner it makes it appear that religion is primarily a set of beliefs, a world view, that may or may not have implications for how we understand and respond to certain kinds of ethical dilemmas. While it is certainly true that Christianity involves beliefs, the character of those beliefs cannot be understood apart from its place in the formation of a community with cultic practices. By focusing on this fact I hope to throw a different perspective on how those who are called to care for the sick can draw upon and count on the particular kind of community we call the church.

I do not intend, for example, to argue that medicine must be reclaimed as in some decisive way dependent on theology. Nor do I want to argue that the development of "medical ethics" will ultimately require the acknowledgment of, or recourse to, theological presuppositions. Rather all I want to try to show is why, given the particular demands put on those who care for the ill, something very much like a church is necessary to sustain that care.

To develop this point I want to call attention to an obvious but often overlooked aspect of illness—namely that when we are sick we hurt and are in pain. I realize that often we are sick and yet not in pain—e.g., hardening of the arteries—but that does not ultimately defeat my general point, since we know that such an illness will lead to physical and mental pain. Nor am I particularly bothered by the observation that many pains are "psychological," having no real physiological basis. Physicians are right to insist that people who say they have pain, even if no organic basis can be found for such pain, are in fact, in pain, though they may be mistaken about what kind of pain it is.

Moreover I am well aware that there are many different kinds of pain, as well as intensity of pains. What is only a minor hurt for me may be a major trauma for someone else. Pain comes in many shapes and sizes and it is never possible to separate the psychological aspects of pain from the organic. For example, suffering, which is not the same as pain since we can suffer without being in pain, is nonetheless akin to pain inasmuch as it is a felt deficiency that can make us as miserable as pain itself.[2]

Yet given these qualifications it remains true that there is a strong connection between pain and illness, an area of our lives in which it is appropriate to call upon the skills of a physician. When we are in pain we want to be helped. But it is exactly at this point that one of the strangest aspects of our being in pain occurs—namely, it is impossible for us to experience one another's pain. That does not mean we cannot communicate to one another our pain. That we can do, but what cannot be done is for you to understand and/or experience my pain as mine.

This puts us under a double burden because we have enough of a problem learning to know one another in the normal aspects of our lives, but when we are in pain our alienation from one another only increases. For no matter how sympathetic we may be to the other in pain, that very pain creates a history and experience that makes the other just that much more foreign to me. Our pains isolate us from one another as they create worlds that cut us off from one another. Consider, for example, the immense gulf between the world of the sick and the healthy. No matter how much we may experience the former, when we are healthy or not in pain we have trouble imagining and understanding the world of the ill.

Indeed the terms we are using are still far too crude. For we do not suffer illness in and of itself, but we suffer this particular kind of illness and have this particular kind of pain. Thus even within the world of illness there are subworlds that are not easily crossed. Think, for example, of how important it is for those suffering from the same illness to share their stories with one another. They do not believe others can understand their particular kind of pain. People with heart disease may find little basis of communion with those suffering from cancer. Pain itself does not create a shared experience; only pain of a particular kind and sort. Moreover the very commonality thus created separates the ill from the healthy in a decisive way.

Pain not only isolates us from one another, but even from ourselves. Think how quickly people with a terribly diseased limb or organ are anxious for surgery in the hope that if it is just cut off or cut out they will not be burdened by the pain that makes them not know themselves. This gangrenous leg is not mine. I would prefer to lose the leg rather than face the reality of its connection to me.

The difficulties pain creates in terms of our relation with ourselves is compounded by the peculiar difficulties it creates for those close to us who do not share our pain. For no matter how sympathetic they may be, no matter how much they may try to be with and comfort us, we know they do not want to experience our pain. I not only cannot, but I do not want to, know the pain you are feeling. No matter how good willed we may be, we cannot take another's pain as our pain. Our pains divide us and there is little we can do to restore our unity.

I suspect this is one of the reasons that chronic illness is such a burden. For often we are willing to be present and sympathetic with someone with an intense but temporary pain—that is, we are willing to be present as long as they work at being "good" sick people who try to get well quickly and do not make too much of their discomfort. We may initially be quite sympathetic with someone with a chronic disease, but it seems to be asking too much of us to be compassionate year in and year out. Thus the universal testimony of people with chronic illness that their illness often results in the alienation of their former friends. This is a problem not only for the person who is ill but also for those closely connected with that person. The family of a person who is chronically ill often discover that the very skills and habits they must learn to be present to the one in pain creates a gulf between themselves and their friends. Perhaps no case illustrates this more poignantly than a family that has a retarded child. Often they discover it is not long before they have a whole new set of friends who also happen to have retarded children [9].

Exactly because pain is so alienating, we are hesitant to admit that we are in pain. To be in pain means we need help, that we are vulnerable to the interests of others, that we are not in control of our destiny. Thus we seek to deny our pain in the hope that we will be able to handle it within ourselves. But the attempt to deal with our pain by ourselves or to deny its existence has the odd effect of only increasing our loneliness. For exactly to the extent I am successful, I create a story about myself that I cannot easily share.

No doubt more can be and needs to be said that would nuance this account of pain and the way it tends to isolate us from one another. Yet I think I have said enough that our attention has been called to this quite common but all the more extraordinary aspect of our existence. Moreover, in the light of this analysis I hope we can now appreciate the remarkable behavior of Job's friends. For in spite of the bad press Job's comforters usually receive (and in many ways it is deserved!), they at least sat on the ground with him for seven days. Moreover they did not speak to him, "for they saw that his suffering was very great." That they did so is truly an act of magnanimity, for most of us are willing to be with sufferers, especially those in such pain that we can hardly recognize them, only if we can "do something" to relieve their suffering or at least distract their attention. Not so with Job's comforters. They sat on the ground with Job doing nothing more than being willing to be present in the face of his suffering.

Now if any of this is close to being right, it puts the task of physicians and others who are pledged to be with the ill in an interesting perspective. For I take it that their activity as physicians is characterized by the fundamental commitment to be, like Job's comforters, in the presence of those who are in pain.[3] At this moment I am not concerned to explore the moral reason for that commitment, but only to note that in fact physicians, nurses, chaplains, and many others are present to the ill as none of the rest of us are. They are the bridge between the world of the ill and the healthy.

Certainly physicians are there because they have been trained with skills that enable them to alleviate the pain of the ill. They have learned from some sick people how to help other sick people. Yet every physician soon learns of the terrible limit of his/her craft, for the sheer particularity of the patient's illness often defies the best knowledge and skill. Even more dramatically, physicians learn that using the best knowledge and skill they have on some patients sometimes has terrible results.

Yet the fact that medicine through the agency of physicians does not and cannot always "cure" in no way qualifies the commitment of the physician. At least it does not do so if we remember that the physician's basic pledge is not to cure, but to care through being present to the one in pain. Yet it is not easy to carry out that commitment on a day-to-day, year-to-year basis. For none of us have the resources to see too much pain without that pain hardening us. Without such a hardening, something we sometimes call by the name of professional distance, we fear we will lose the ability to feel at all.

Yet the physician cannot help but be touched and, thus, tainted by the world of the sick. Through their willingness to be present to us in our most vulnerable moments they are forever scarred with our pain — a pain that we the healthy want to deny or at least keep at arm's length. They have seen a world we do not want to see until it is forced on us, and we will accept them into polite community only to the extent they keep that world hidden from us. But when we are driven into that world we want to be able to count on their skill and their presence, even though we have been unwilling to face that reality while we were healthy.

But what do these somewhat random and controversial observations have to do with helping us better understand the relation between medicine and the church and/or the story of my boyhood friendship with Bob? To begin with the latter, I think in some ways the mechanism that was working during that trying time with Bob is quite similar to the mechanism that works on a day-to-day basis in medicine. For the physician, and others concerned with our illness, are called to be present during times of great pain and tragedy. Indeed physicians, because of their moral commitments, have the privilege and the burden to be with us when we are most vulnerable. The physician learns our deepest fears and our profoundest hopes. As patients, that is also why so often we fear the physician, because she/he may know us better than we know ourselves. Surely that is one of the reasons that confidentially is so crucial to the patient-physician relation, since it is a situation of such intimacy.

But just to the extent that the physician has been granted the privilege of being with us while we are in pain, that very experience creates the seeds of distrust and fear. We are afraid of one another's use of the knowledge gained, but even more deeply we fear remembering the pain as part of our history. Thus every crisis that joins us in a common fight for health also has the potential for separating us more profoundly after the crisis. Yet the physician is pledged to come to our aid again and again, no matter how we may try to protect ourselves from his/her presence.

The physician, on the other hand, has yet another problem, for how can anyone be present to the ill day in and day out without learning to dislike, if not positively detest, our smallness in the face of pain. People in pain are omnivorous in their appetite for help, and they will use us up if we let them. Fortunately the physician has other patients who can give him distance from any patient who requires too much. But the problem still remains how morally those who are pledged to be with the ill never lose their ability to see the humanity that our very suffering often comes close to obliterating. For the physician cannot, as Bob and I did, drift apart and away from those whom he or she is pledged to serve. At least they cannot if I am right that medicine is first of all pledged to be nothing more than a human presence in the face of suffering.

But how can we account for such a commitment — the commitment to be present to those in pain? No doubt basic human sympathy is not to be discounted, but it does not seem to be sufficient to account for a group of people dedicated to being present to the ill as their vocation in life. Nor does it seem sufficient to account for the acquiring of the skills necessary to sustain that presence in a manner that is not alienating and the source of distrust in a community.

To learn how to be present in that way we need examples — that is, a people who have so learned to embody such a presence in their lives that it has become the marrow of their habits. The church at least claims to be such a community, as it is a group of people called out by a God who, we believe, is always present to us, both in our sin and our faithfulness. Because of God's faithfulness we are supposed to be a people who have learned how to be faithful to one another by our willingness to be present, with all our vulnerabilities, to one another. For what does our God require of us other than our unfailing presence in the midst of the world's sin and pain? Thus our willingness to be ill and to ask for help, as well as our willingness to be present with the ill is no special or extraordinary activity, but a form of the Christian obligation to be present to one another in and out of pain.

Moreover, it is such a people who should have learned how to be present with those in pain without that pain driving them further apart. For the very bond that pain forms between us becomes the basis for alienation, as we have no means to know how to make it part of our common history. Just as it is painful to remember our sins, so we seek not to remember our pain, since we desire to live as if our world and existence were a pain-free one. Only a people trained in remembering, and remembering as a communal act, their sins and pains can offer a paradigm for sustaining across time a painful memory so that it acts to heal rather than to divide.

Thus medicine needs the church not to supply a foundation for its moral commitments, but rather as a resource of the habits and practices necessary to sustain the care of those in pain over the long haul. For it is no easy matter to be with the ill, especially when we cannot do much for them other than simply be present. Our very helplessness too often turns to hate, both toward the one in pain and ourselves, as we despise them for reminding us of our helplessness. Only when we remember that our presence is our doing, when sitting on the ground seven days saying nothing is what we can do, can we be saved from our fevered and hopeless attempt to control others' and our own existence. Of course to believe that such presence is what we can and should do entails a belief in a presence in and beyond this world. And it is certainly true many today no longer believe in or experience such a presence. If that is the case, then I do wonder if medicine as an activity of presence is possible in a world without God.

Another way of raising this issue is to ask the relation between prayer and medical care. Nothing I have said about the basic pledge of physicians to be present to the ill entails that they should not try to develop the skills necessary to help those in pain and illness. Certainly they should, as theirs is an art that is one of our most valuable resources for the care of one another. But no matter how powerful that craft becomes, it cannot in principle rule out the necessity of prayer. For prayer is not a supplement to the insufficiency of our medical knowledge and practice; nor is it some divine insurance policy that our medical skill will work; rather, our prayer is the means that we have to make God present whether our medical skill is successful or not. So understood, the issue is not whether medical care and prayer are antithetical, but how medical care can ever be sustained without the necessity of continued prayer.

Finally, those involved in medicine need the church as otherwise they cannot help but be alienated from the rest of us. For unless there is a body of people who have learned the skills of presence, the world of the ill cannot help but become a separate world both for the ill and/or those who care for them. Only a community that is pledged not to fear the stranger—and illness always makes us a stranger to ourselves and others—can welcome the continued presence of the ill in our midst. The hospital is, after all, first and foremost a house of hospitality along the way of our journey with finitude. It is our sign that we will not abandon those who have become ill simply because they currently are suffering the sign of that finitude. If the hospital, as too often is the case today, becomes but a means of isolating the ill from the rest of us, then we have betrayed its central purpose and distorted our community and ourselves.

If the church can be the kind of people who show clearly that they have learned to be with the sick and the dying, it may just be that through that process we will better understand the relation of salvation to health, religion to medicine. Or perhaps even more, we will better understand what kind of medicine we ought to practice, since too often we try to substitute doing for presence. It is surely the case, as Paul Ramsey reminds us, "that not since Socrates posed the question have we learned how to teach virtue. The quandaries of medical ethics are not unlike that question. Still, we can no longer rely upon the ethical assumptions in our culture to be powerful enough or clear enough to instruct the profession in virtue; therefore the medical profession should no longer believe that the personal integrity of physicians alone is enough; neither can anyone count on values being transmitted without thought" ([14], p. xviii). All I have tried to do is remind us that neither can we count on such values being transmitted without a group of people who believe in and live trusting in God's unfailing presence.

NOTES

1. Ramsey's position is complex and I certainly cannot do it justice here. His emphasis on "love transforming natural law" would tend to qualify the point made above. Yet it is also true that Ramsey's increasing use of covenant language has gone hand in hand with his readiness to identify certain "covenants" that need no "transformation." Of course he could object that the covenant between doctor and patient is the result of Christian love operating in history.

2. For a fuller account of the complex relation between pain and suffering see [11].

3. I am indebted to a conversation with Dr. Earl Shelp for helping me understand better the significance of this point.

REFEREENCES

[1] Amundsen, D., and Ferngren, G. 1982. "Medicine and Religion: Pre-Christian Antiquity." In M. Marty and K. Vaux, eds., *Health/Medicine and the Faith Traditions*, 53-92. Philadelphia: Fortress Press.

[2] Amundsen, D., and Ferngren, G. 1982. "Medicine and Religion: Early Christianity Through the Middle Ages." In M. Marty and K. Vaux, eds., *Health/Medicine and the Faith Traditions*, 93-132.

[3] Childress, J. 1981. *Priorities in Biomedical Ethics*. Philadelphia: Westminster Press.

[4] Curran, C. 1978. *Issues in Sexual and Medical Ethics*. Notre Dame, Ind.: University of Notre Dame Press.

[5] Fletcher, J. 1954. *Morals and Medicine*. Boston: Beacon Press.

[6] Gustafson, J. 1975. *The Contributions of Theology to Medical Ethics*. Milwaukee: Marquette University Press.

[7] Haring, B. 1973. *Medical Ethics*. South Bend, Ind.: Fides Publishers.

[8] Hauerwas, S. 1983. "On Keeping Theological Ethics Theological." In A. MacIntyre and S. Hauerwas, eds., *Revisions: Changing Perspectives in Moral Philosophy*, 16-42. Notre Dame, Ind.: University of Notre Dame Press.

[9] Hauerwas, S. 1982. "The Retarded, Society and the Family: The Dilemma of Care." In S. Hauerwas, ed., *Responsibility for Devalued Persons*. Springfield, Ill.: Charles C. Thomas. Reprinted in the present volume (see essay no. 11).

[10] Hauerwas S. 1982. "Authority and the Profession of Medicine." In G., Agich, *Responsibility in Health Care*, 83-104. Dordrecht, Holland: Reidel. Reprinted in the present volume (see essay no. 2).

[11] Hauerwas, S. 1979. "Reflections on Suffering, Death, and Medicine," *Ethics in Science and Medicine* 6: 229-237. Reprinted in the present volume (see essay no. 1).

[12] MacIntyre. A. 1981. "Can Medicine Dispense with a Theological Perspective on Human Nature?" In D. Callahan and H. Engelhardt, eds., *The Roots of Ethics*, 119-138. New York: Plenum Press.

[13] Ramsey, P. 1973. "The Nature of Medical Ethics." In R. Neatch, M. Gaylin, and C. Morgan, eds., *The Teaching of Medical Ethics*, 14-28. Hastings-on-Hudson, N.Y.: Hastings Center.

[14] Ramsey, P. 1970. *The Patient as Person*. New Haven: Yale University Press.

PART TWO

Theological Reflections on Living, Dying, and Experimentation

4

Religious Concepts of Brain Death
and Associated Problems

The Limits of Theological Determination of the Moment of Death

Theologians are considered to be an odd lot today. We sense the public's bemusement as soon as we try to explain what we do, because we are immediately subject to suspicious questioning. If you are fortunate, your listener misunderstands theology for geology and assumes you are engaged in an honest endeavor. However, if you go on to explain that you are not a geologist, but a theologian, you are confronted with a quizzical stare that makes you feel that an explanation, if not an apology, is in order. Generally, I assume that this means that people do not think it odd for someone to spend his or her life thinking about rocks, but that it is an aberration to spend your life thinking about God.

There is, of course, good reason for this judgment—thinking about rocks seems to have some payoff in a way that thinking about God does not. Rocks are connected to oil in an immediate and direct way, and even the best prayer will not make a car run without gas. Therefore, when theologians are invited to speak at conferences on such matters as the determination of brain death, they are extremely anxious to please. Such conferences represent an opportunity to show that theology has concrete relevance.

Therefore you will understand how disappointed I am to have to tell you that there is nothing in Christian convictions that would entail preference for one definition of death over another. That is not to say that there have not been a lot of perceptive and incisive things said by theologians about the determination of the moment of death. However, it remains unclear what connection there is between their theological views and their judgments about death.

The claim that a connection must be demonstrated between Chris-

87

tian conviction and determination of the moment of death may seem odd. After all, physicians often deal with people who tell them that their Christian convictions have something to do with their death. There seems to be good reason for this claim, since basic biblical texts deal with death. Thus in Paul's letter to the Romans we are told

> If we have died with Christ, we believe that we shall also live with him. For we know that Christ being raised from the dead will never die again; death no longer has dominion over him. The death he died he died to sin, once for all, but the life he lives he lives to God. So you also must consider yourselves dead to sin and alive to God in Christ. (Romans 6:8–11)

In even more ringing terms Paul says

> Who shall separate us from the love of Christ? Shall tribulation or distress or persecution or famine, or nakedness, or peril, or sword? As it is written, "For thy sake we are being killed all the day long; we are regarded as sheep to be slaughtered." No, in all these things we are more than conquerors through him who loved us. For I am sure that neither death, nor life, nor angels, nor principalities, nor things present, nor things to come, nor powers, nor height, nor depth, nor anything else in all creation, will be able to separate us from the love of God in Christ Jesus our Lord. (Romans 8:35–39)

These are powerful and substantive claims. Yet Paul Ramsey, a theologian who has dealt extensively with death and dying, stated with regard to a theological definition of the moment of death that "a theologian or moralist as such knows nothing about such questions; the determination of death is a medical matter; and a theologian or moralist can offer only his reflections upon the meaning of respect for life and of care of the dying, and issue some warnings of the moral complexities surrounding such matters" ([8], p. 104).

In this essay I will explain why Ramsey is right to deny that there is a theological definition of the moment of death. Christians hold some very substantive beliefs about death itself, however, and I want to suggest how in general those beliefs help to provide a framework for the moral and practical considerations connected with definitions of the moment of death. In the foregoing passages from Paul death is described theologically and morally. I will try to show *how* those perspectives on death help to set the kind of questions that should be asked about the meaning and status of any proposed definition of the moment of death.

The Meaning and Status of Brain Death

In order to understand the reluctance of theologians to provide a "religious concept of brain death," it is necessary to be clear about what brain death means. There is no reason for me to go over the work that Veatch [9] has done so well, but I will center my concerns about the very helpful distinction he provides. Veatch's central point is that the concept of death should not be confused with the criteria that determine when death has occurred. He rightly argues that the concept of death involves a philosophical judgment of a significant change that has happened in a person. Thus the concept of death is a correlative of what one takes to be the necessary condition of human life, e.g., the capacity for bodily integration or the potential for consciousness.

Correlative to different concepts of death are certain loci and criteria of death. Loci are places where we look to determine whether or not the person is dead, i.e., heart, brain, neocortex. The criteria of death are those empirical measurements that can be made to determine whether a person is dead, such as cessation of respiration or a flat EEG. The subtle point in Veatch's analysis is that there is no necessary connection between certain concepts of death and the determination of the locus and criteria of death ([9], p. 51). Rather, the claim is made that certain associations of the loci and criteria of death with certain concepts of death seem more appropriate than others, but these associations are pragmatic and contingent, not conceptual and necessary. Thus it seems reasonable to identify the locus of death with the brain if one understands the concept of death to involve the irreversible loss of the capacity for bodily integration. It also seems appropriate to use the criteria of the Harvard report as an indication of when death has occurred. "Brain death" is an empirical standard for verifying a death, but it does not involve one and only one concept of death. So Veatch is right to suggest that "terms such as brain death or heart death should be avoided because they tend to obscure the fact we are searching for the meaning of death of the person as a whole" ([9], p. 37).

For those dealing with dying patients this kind of analysis may

seem to be question-begging. However, such an analysis is but a reminder that genuinely practical matters often raise deep theoretical
issues. These issues are absolutely crucial if we are to consider questions such as how to determine the moment of death without confusing them with questions concerning the worth of prolonging life under
certain circumstances. For nothing could be more dangerous than the
attempt to substitute a definition of the moment of death for a moral
question concerning our obligation to keep ourselves and others alive
under conditions of distress. A definition of death should not preclude
the question of the worth of a life. The question regarding the worth
of Karen Quinlan's life should not be precluded by defining her as dead.

This distinction helps to clarify why the issue of defining the
criteria of death should not be determined in terms of the need for
transplant organs. Whatever the concept of death we think appropriate,
the criteria of death should take into account the dying person's needs.
If the phrase "right to die" makes any sense at all, it should at least
mean that we should be allowed to die without the meaning of our
death being determined by someone else's needs.

More important for the purpose of this paper, however, is the
distinction between the concept of death and the loci and criteria of
death to help make clear the role of Christian convictions about death.
As I suggested, there may not be a religious concept of brain death.
That does not mean, though, that Christian beliefs may not contribute
to an understanding of the concept of death. This issue has been confused in the past by assuming that the use of a metaphor like the "heart"
in religious discourse implied a position about the locus or criteria of
death. But "heart" so used is not an empirical description of a part
of the body, but rather an indication of the whole person's engage-
ment with life. Thus the question arises of how Christian beliefs about
the nature of death might make a difference in how the concept of
death is understood.

Sacredness of Life and the Concept of Death

The claim that Christian convictions make a difference in how
the concept of death is understood remains ambiguous. Note how
abstract such phrases as "irreversible loss of the soul from the body,"
or "irreversible loss of capacity for bodily integration," or "loss of con-

sciousness" are when compared with the life plans of people. For example, I have known some "good old boys" who felt strongly that when you became too old to ride a horse you might as well be dead. If you told them that they were thereby committed to assuming death to consist of "loss of consciousness," thereby making the neocortex the locus of death and the criterion a flat EEG, they would probably tell you that they don't give a damn.

Christian beliefs about death work like "riding a horse," i.e., the beliefs shape the Christian's conception of death. The Christian is concerned not with life as an end in itself, but rather as the medium for service in God's kingdom. Put differently, no one lives just to live. We each live for some purpose or purposes. These purposes set certain boundaries that determine the meaning and significance of death. Christians believe that their lives have been determined by the purposes of God as manifest in the history of Israel and Jesus' cross and resurrection. Thus for Paul the "death" that concerns him the most is the death that reigns in this life through the power of sin. The problem is that there is no clear inference that can be drawn from this sense of the purpose of life concerning which concept of death is most appropriate for the Christian.

With respect to life, however, it has recently been claimed that the basic stance of Christians toward life is that it is sacred. This obviously has been claimed in questions concerning death and dying and abortions. There is surely much about the phrase "sanctity of life" in which Christians have a stake. We believe that God has sanctified every living thing and that each of his creatures, even the most wayward, cannot escape his care — in both life and death.

This claim regarding the sacredness of life often indicates the refusal of the Christian to separate the spirit from the body. Although there is much talk about the soul in Christian discourse, Christians always maintain the Jewish sense of the body's significance. Thus Ramsey maintains that

> Just as man is sacredness in the social and political order, so he is a sacredness in the natural, biological order. He is a sacredness in bodily life. He is a person who within the ambience of the flesh claims our care. He is an embodied soul or ensouled body. He is therefore a sacredness in illness and in his dying. . . . The sanctity of human life prevents ultimate trespass upon him even for the sake of treating his bodily life,

> or for the sake of others who are also only a sacredness in their bodily
> lives. ([8], p. xiii)

This at least means that Christians will be suspicious of any concept
of death that associates the death only with the so-called "higher forms
of our life." Of course that does not mean that the neocortex is ruled
out as the locus of death, since it may well be the best indication that
the bodily conditions necessary for our consciousness can no longer
be sustained.

It is a mistake to assume that "sanctity of life" is a sufficient
criterion for an appropriate concept of death. Appeals to the sanctity
of life beg exactly the question at issue, namely, that you know what
kind of life it is that should be treated as sacred. More troubling for
me, however, is how the phrase "sanctity of life," when separated from
its theological context, became an ideological slogan for a narrow individualism antithetical to the Christian way of life. Put starkly, Christians are not fundamentally concerned about living. Rather, their concern is to die for the right thing. Appeals to the sanctity of life as an
ideology make it appear that Christians are committed to the proposi-
tion that there is nothing in life worth dying for.

When this happens Christians unwittingly embody the modern
view that death is the one thing we can be sure about in life and that
it is to be avoided as long as possible. As my former colleague, Rev.
John Dunne, C.S.C., has pointed out, Descartes said "I think, therefore
I am," while modern man says "I am going to die, therefore I am."
Our identity is no longer anchored in life, but in death. As a result,
death becomes the overriding enemy. But such an attitude is antithetical
to the Christian belief that our identity is anchored in God's love as
revealed in the cross. Even death itself cannot separate us from that.

Thus the phrase "sanctity of life," when used as an ideology,
dangerously suggests that for a Christian life is an end in itself. Our
sacredness rests then on something such as rationality. But as Ramsey
has suggested

> one grasps the religious outlook upon the sanctity of human life only
> if he sees that this life is asserted to be surrounded by sanctity that need
> not be in man; that the most dignity a man ever possesses is a dignity
> that is alien to him. . . . The value of a human life is ultimately
> grounded in the value God is placing on it. Anyone who can himself
> stand imaginatively even for a moment with an outlook where everything

is referred finally to God — who, from things that are not, brings into being things that are — should be able to see that God's deliberation about the man need have only begun. ([7], p. 11-12)

Therefore life for Christians is not sacred in the strict sense. Christians view life as a gift, but a gift for which they must care [2]. Thus the claim that life is sacred is not really so much a statement about ourselves as it is an indication of the kind of respect that we owe our neighbor. Our life and the lives of our neighbors are to be protected, since they are not ours to dispose of. For our dying as much as our living should be determined by our conviction that we are not our own.

But what do these homiletical flourishes have to do with the concept of death? They at least make clear why Christians have an aversion to the connotation of hastened death associated with the unhappy word *euthanasia* [2]. However, these considerations also help us understand why Christians, in spite of their condemnation of euthanasia, have assumed that death need not be prolonged in all cases. This distinction between ordinary and extraordinary means of prolonging life, a distinction that is probably more trouble than it is worth, was the result of Christians' attempt to balance their sense that their lives were not at their disposal with their sense that death is not to be opposed unconditionally. Veatch is right to suggest that reflection on the right to refuse treatment is a much better means to consider such questions ([9], pp. 116–163).

Moreover, Ramsey has argued that the question of "updating the criteria" of death in the context of Christian convictions is better described as an attempt to develop a criterion for when to use a respirator ([8], p. 81). I think it is useful to note why Ramsey thinks he has a theological stake in describing the issue in this manner. He fears that "brain death" might be taken to indicate that a person's primary value is determined by intelligence rather than by his or her existence as one of God's children. Thus he can argue that the criteria of "brain death" are not essentially different from "heart death" criteria, but rather denote a procedural difference that has come about because of the extensive use of life-supporting techniques ([8], p. 87). Ramsey therefore has no objection to the criteria of death suggested by the Harvard report, since he assumes that the heart and lungs can only function artifically when there is total brain death. Thus there is no moral or theological commitment to continue using a respirator in such a case.

However, it would seem that Ramsey would have difficulty approving the definition of brain death as a "dead" neocortex accompanied by a brain stem still capable of maintaining heart and lung function. I mention this because Veatch has argued that, all other things being equal, the death of the neocortex should be sufficient to indicate that death should be declared. There are, of course, empirical issues involved in this proposal (i.e., whether an EEG unfailingly predicts the irreversible loss of consciousness associated with the death of the neocortex). My concern, however, is whether or not there is any theological issue at stake in this difference between Ramsey and Veatch.

Ramsey might well suggest that Veatch assumes that the value of human life is only related to our consciousness and capacity for social interaction, and thus fails to see that the value of life should primarily be determined by God. However, this kind of argument assumes that there is a strong logical connection between the criteria of death and the concept and correlative worth of life. Veatch is not saying that the value of life is associated only with consciousness, but rather that consciousness is the necessary condition for any values. Moreover, Veatch's concern is primarily practical. His question is whether there are any indications that might help us to know when not to subject those who are dying to a mercy grown cruel through the power of our technology. While it is cruel not to try to sustain life, it may be just as cruel to extend care unconditionally. Interestingly, it is in terms of these practical issues that Christian convictions may be the most relevant.

The Christian Way of Death

With respect to the practical issues surrounding the care of the dying I now want to provide a slightly different perspective. Briefly, I want to suggest that we have had trouble considering how we should care for the dying because we have not thought enough about what kind of responsibilities the one who is dying should have. In other words, the moral street here is not one way—the dying person has obligations to the living that are important for us to understand in the care of the dying. The attempt to determine the moment of death may be an attempt to avoid determining when it is time to die.

Today there is much talk about learning to care for the dying.

Generally this means that the patient ought to be regarded as primary, that he or she is someone to whom something terrible is happening and that we ought to help if we can. The assumption is that death, like a serious illness, robs persons of almost all claims to moral agency. The primary issue, then, is embodied in the question of the kind of care we ought to give someone so struck.

Also, the admonition that we must learn to care for the dying is an attempt to recover the more personal side of medicine. What the dying often need is not further medical care, especially if that care is used only to prolong the dying process; but it is claimed that the patient needs personal care. Care is not synonymous with cure and it is argued that the doctor and nurses should help the patient in a psychological and moral way. These admonitions to learn how to care for the dying are salutary, but they assume that the care of the dying is primarily concerned with the attitudes of the living toward what is essentially a passive object.

However, as Milton Mayeroff has reminded us, care must be extended in such a manner that the one cared for is given the freedom to care also:

> To care for another person, in the most significant sense, is to help him grow and actualize himself. Consider, for example, a father caring for his child. He respects the child as existing in his own right and as striving to grow. Caring is the antithesis of simply using the other person to satisfy one's own needs. Caring, as helping another grow and actualize himself, is a process, a way of relating to someone that involves development, in the same way that friendship can only emerge in time through mutual trust and a deepening and qualitative transformation of the relationship. ([6], p. 1)

This sense of caring cannot help but strike us as a little odd when it comes to caring for the dying, because the dying seem to be ending their growing. Interestingly, we have recently come up with an answer to this problem. We can help the one who is dying to accept his or her death in the manner suggested by Kübler-Ross [5]. We are thus engaged in the extremely odd enterprise of encouraging people to die better than they have lived. No one can die angry or apathetically because it becomes imperative that we all die with a quiet, brave acceptance.

There are some deep problems associated with this kind of proposal. By transforming her descriptive stages into normative recommendations, Dr. Ross runs the risk of developing an extraordinarily manipulative strategy to deal with dying. More importantly, there is nothing associated with Christian beliefs that should require us to want our death. However, these beliefs do make a great deal of difference with respect to our learning how to die.

It is clear from the passages from Paul cited at the beginning of this paper that death is not the worst thing that could happen to a Christian. But neither is it a good thing. According to Paul, a Christian may desire death in a manner which denotes lack of trust in God's triumph over death. Death is both a friend and enemy. It is a friend in that without it we would not be forced to value one thing in life over another. Ironically, death creates the economy that makes life worthwhile. But because death is a friend it also becomes our enemy, for what we come to value and love we want to continue to value and love [3].

Moreover, the language associated with the acceptance of death must be carefully used. If the one who is dying accepts death too well, it plays a cruel trick on the living. One who is too willing to die can make us feel that our own lack of care caused the one who died to leave life without wishing to retain anything. (Of course, we are talking here about a gradual rather than a sudden or accidental death.)

It is important, then, that the one who is dying exercise the responsibility to die well. That is, the person should die in a manner that is morally commensurate with the kind of trust that has sustained him or her in life. In terms of the language that I used earlier, it means that we should die in such a manner that others see that they are sustaining us and that correlatively due credit is given to God as the ultimate giver of life.

The very idea we should take responsibility for how we die may strike many as odd. That such is the case is but an indication of our society's general attitude toward death. For example most people when asked how they want to die say in their sleep or suddenly—i.e., in a manner that they do not have to prepare for their dying. In contrast medieval people most feared sudden death since such a death would prevent from preparing for their death both in terms of their social responsibilities and their eternal destiny. Thus they preferred death in battle, since they had time before hand to prepare, and cancer was not for them the dreaded disease it is for us. The necessity we feel to define the "moment of death" is partly the result of our attempt to avoid preparing for death and thus making the moment of our death unexpected.

Thus the concern to recapture the meaning of "natural death" is salutary. Daniel Callahan has recently tried to define natural death as when (1) one's life work has been accomplished; (2) one's moral obligations to those for whom one has responsibilities have been discharged; (3) one's death will not seem to others an offense to sense or sensibility, or will not tempt others to despair and rage at human existence; and (4) one's process of dying is not marked by unbearable and degrading pain [1].

Callahan notes that all four points are filled with ambiguity (e.g., it makes a lot of difference how you conceive your life's work and whom you think you have responsibilities to) and that it is hard to die without offending someone. However, there is much to commend Callahan's suggestion. As Eberhard Jungel has argued, the Christian conviction that we have been freed from the curse of death by Jesus Christ implies that

> human life has a natural end which comes when the time allotted to life has expired. Man has a right to die this death and no other. One of the duties of Christian faith is to see that this right is recognized. There is therefore an immediate connection between the proclamation of the death of Jesus Christ and the concern that man should have the right to die a natural death. ([4], p. 132)

There are a couple of qualifications that need to be made with respect to Jungel's and Callahan's defense of the idea of "natural death." First, we should avoid the phrase "right to die." The term is unclear and Callahan observes that no society can guarantee that there will be no "deaths of the kind that lead people to fear their own death, or wonder about the rationality and benignness of the universe" [1]. Secondly, I suspect that the phrase "natural death" is too misleading to be of much help. In a sense no death is natural, but is, as Veatch suggests, the result of some human choices. To perpetuate the fiction of "natural death" may give us the feeling that we are relieved of responsibility, but it does so at the "expense of continuing the suffering of death striking out in random and unregulated viciousness. . . . [Natural death] is the death of the animal species, but in being so it is subhuman. If man is a responsible agent charged with the task of creating and sustaining his life and his environment, then such fictions are escapist. Such fiction may give freedom, but the result is tyranny. To escape from responsibility to the imagined comforts of natural death cannot be a sustainable defense" ([9], p. 302).

It seems to me, however, that Callahan's proposal does not hinge on a notion of natural death, but is really an attempt to indicate what an acceptable or perhaps even a good death would entail. A good death is a death that we can prepare for through living because we are able to see that death is but a necessary correlative to a good life. Thus a good death is not natural in the sense that it may well occur before our natural machinery runs down, but it is good if it is commensurate with those commitments that sustained our life. For Christians this means that while we do not wish to die, we do not oppose death as if life were an end in itself. For as Augustine said, "Death is [to not] love God, and that is when we prefer anything to Him in affection and pursuit."

Finally, what do these kinds of concerns have to do with the issue of brain death? They remind us that "brain death" does not function just as a locus of death, but as a symbol of when it is time to die. But I am suggesting that if we are to die a good death, we must not allow the symbol of brain death to tyrannize us by requiring that we delay death so long that we can no longer die a good death. "Brain death" may well serve as an indication of when the living are released from certain claims having to do with care of the dying, but it should not be used as a substitute for the responsibility each of us has to die our own death. "Brain death" or "heart death" should not remove the responsibility and risk that are the necessary concomitants of our willingness to die a good death.

REFERENCES

[1] Callahan, Daniel. 1977. "On Defining 'Natural Death.'" *Hastings Center Report* 7, no. 3: 32-37.
[2] Hauerwas, Stanley. 1977. *Truthfulness and Tragedy: Further Investigation in Christian Ethics*. Notre Dame, Ind.: University of Notre Dame Press. See especially pp. 101-115.
[3] Hauerwas, Stanley, 1974. *Vision and Virtue: Essays in Christian Ethical Reflection*. Notre Dame, Ind.: Fides Press; rpt. University of Notre Dame Press, 1981. See especially pp. 166-186.

[4] Jungel, Eberhard. 1974. *Death: The Riddle and the Mystery*. Philadelphia: Westminster.

[5] Kübler-Ross, E. 1969. *On Death and Dying*. New York: Macmillan.

[6] Mayeroff, Milton. 1971. *On Caring*. New York: Harper and Row.

[7] Ramsey, Paul. 1971 "The Morality of Abortion." In James Rachels, ed., *Moral Problems*. New York: Harper and Row.

[8] Ramsey, Paul. 1970. *The Patient as Person*. New Haven: Yale University Press. See especially pp. 59-164.

[9] Veatch, Robert. 1976. *Death, Dying and the Biological Revolution: Our Last Quest for Responsibility*. New Haven: Yale University Press.

5

Rational Suicide and Reasons for Living

Suicide and the Ethics of Autonomy

There is a peculiar ambiguity concerning the morality of suicide in our society. Our commitment to the autonomy of the individual at least implies that suicide may not only be rational, but a "right."[1] Yet many continue to believe that people attempting suicide must be sick and therefore prevented from killing themselves. This ambiguity makes us hesitant even to analyze the morality of suicide because we fear we may discover that our society lacks any coherent moral policy or basis for preventing suicide.

Therefore the very idea of "rational suicide" is a bit threatening. We must all feel a slight twinge of concern about the book published by the British Voluntary Euthanasia Society that describes the various painless and foolproof methods of suicide. But it is by no means clear why we feel uncomfortable about having this kind of book widely distributed. As Nicholas Reed, the general secretary of the Society, suggests: suicide is "more and more seen as an acceptable way for a life to end, vastly preferable to some long, slow, painful death. We're simply helping in the fight for another human right—the right to die" (*New York Times*, 1980: A18).

We think there must be something wrong with this, but we are not sure what. I suspect our unease about these matters is part of the reason we wish to deny the existence of rational or autonomous suicide. If all potential suicides can be declared ill by definition, then we can prevent them (ironically) because the agent lacks autonomy. Therefore we intervene to prevent suicides in the name of autonomy, which, if we were consistent, should require us to consider suicide a permissible moral act.

Once I was a participant in a seminar in medical ethics at one of our most prestigious medical schools. I was there to speak about suicide, but the week before, the seminar had considered abortion. At that time I was told by these beginning medical students they de-

100

cided it was their responsibility to perform an abortion if a woman requested it because a woman has the right to determine what she should do with her body — a conclusion that they felt was clearly ethically justified on grounds of protecting the autonomy of the patient. Moreover, this position, they argued, was appropriate if the professional dominance and paternalism of the medical profession was to be broken.

However, I asked them what they would do if they were attending in the emergency room and someone was brought in with slashed wrists with a suicide note pinned to his shirt front. First of all, would they take the time to read the note to discover the state of the patient? Secondly, would they say this is clearly not a medical matter and refuse to accept the patient? Or would they immediately begin to save the person's life? With the same unanimity concerning their responsibility to perform abortion, they felt they must immediately begin trying to save the person's life.

The reason they gave to justify their intervention was that anyone taking his or her life must surely be sick. But it was not clear what kind of "sickness" was under consideration, unless we define life itself as some kind of syndrome. Failing to make the case that all suicides must be sick, they then suggested they must act to save such a person's life because it was their responsibility as doctors. But again I pressed them on what right they had to impose their role-related responsibilities on those who did not seek their services and, in fact, had clearly tried to avoid coming in contact with them. They then appealed to experience, citing cases when people have recovered from suicide attempts only to be thankful they had been helped. But again such appeals are not convincing, since we can also point to the many who are not happy about being saved and soon make another attempt.

Our discussion began to be more and more frustrating for all involved, so a compromise was suggested. These future physicians felt the only solution was that when a suicide came to the emergency room the first time that doctor's responsibility must always be to save the life. However a person who came in a second time could be allowed to die. That kind of solution, however, is not only morally unsatisfactory, but pragmatically difficult to institutionalize. What if each time the person was brought to the hospital a different physician was present.

I have told this story because I think it nicely illustrates the kind of difficulties we feel when we try to get a moral handle on suicide. We feel that Beauchamp and Childress are right that if suicide is *gen-*

uinely autonomous and there are no powerful utilitarian "reasons of human worth and dignity standing in the way, then we ought to allow the person to commit suicide, because we would otherwise be violating the person's autonomy" ([4], p. 93).

However I want to suggest that this way of putting the matter, while completely consistent with an ethics of autonomy, is also deeply misleading. It is misleading not only because it reveals the insufficiency of autonomy either as a basis or ideal for the moral life ([5] and [6]), but also it simply fails to provide an appropriate account of why any of us decide or should decide to stay alive. Indeed it is odd to think of our willingness to live as a decision. For example, Beauchamp and Childress do not explain how anyone could take account of *all* relevant variables and future possibilities in considering suicide. That seems far too strong a demand, for if we required it of even our most important decisions it would stop us from acting at all.

Yet by challenging the claim that autonomous suicide is morally acceptable I want clearly to distinguish my position from those who are intent to deny the possibility of rational suicide. I think that suicide can be and often is a rational decision of an "autonomous" agent, but I do not therefore think it is justified. It is extremely interesting, for example, that Augustine did not claim that suicide was irrational in criticizing the Stoics' acceptance and even recommendation of suicide. Rather he pointed out that their acceptance of suicide belied their own understanding of the relation between evil and happiness and how a wise man thus should deal with adversity. Though the quote is long I think it worth providing the full text. Augustine says,

> There is a mighty force in the evils which compel a man, and, according to those philosophers, even a wise man, to rob himself of his existence as a man; although they say, and say with truth, that the first and greatest utterance of nature, as we may call it, is that a man should be reconciled to himself and for that reason should naturally shun death — that he should be his own friend, in that he should emphatically desire to continue as a living being and to remain alive in this combination of body and soul, and that this should be his aim. There is a mighty force in those evils which overpower this natural feeling which makes us employ all our strength in our endeavor to avoid death — which defeat this feeling so utterly that what was shunned is now wished and longed for, and, if it cannot come to him from some other source, is inflicted on a man by himself. There is a mighty force in those evils

which make Fortitude a murderer—if indeed she is still to be called fortitude when she is so utterly vanquished by those evils that she not only cannot by her endurance keep guard over the man she has undertaken to govern and protect, but is herself compelled to go so far as to kill him. The wise man ought, indeed, to endure even death with a steadfastness, but a death that comes to him from outside himself. Whereas if he is compelled, as those philosophers say, to inflict it on himself, they must surely admit that these are not only evils, but intolerable evils, when they compel him to commit this crime.

It follows from this that the life weighed down by such great and grievous ills, or at the mercy of such chances, would never be called happy, if the men who so term it, and who, when overcome by the growing weights of ills, surrender to adversity compassing their own death—if these people would bring themselves to surrender to the truth, when overcome by sound reasoning, in their quest for the happy life, and would give up supposing that the ultimate, Supreme God is something to be enjoyed by them in this condition of mortality. ([1], pp. 856-857)

The question is not, therefore, the question of whether suicide is "rational." Augustine knew well that the Stoics could provide outstanding examples of cool, unemotional, and rational suicide. He rather asks what kind of blessedness we should expect out of life. For Augustine the Stoic approval of suicide was an indication of the insufficient account they provided about what human existence should be about—namely, they failed to see that the only happiness worth desiring is that which comes from friendship with the true God. "Yet" he says, "these philosophers refuse to believe in this blessedness because they do not see it; and so they attempt to fabricate for themselves an utterly delusive happiness by means of a virtue whose falsity is in proportion to its arrogance" ([1], p. 857).[2] So the issue, if Augustine is right as I believe him to be, is how suicide is understood within a conception of life we think good and worthy.

The Grammar of Suicide

Before developing this line of reasoning, however, it should be pointed out that the discussion to this point has been trading on the assumption that we know what suicide is. Yet that is simply not the case. For as Beauchamp and Childress suggest, definitions of suicide such as "an intentionally caused self-destruction not forced by the action of another person" are not nearly as unambiguous as they may at first seem. For example they point out when persons suffering from a terminal illness or mortal injury allow their death to occur we find ourselves reluctant to call that act "suicide," but if persons with a terminal illness take their life by active means we do refer to that act as one of suicide. Yet to only describe those acts that involve a direct action as suicide is misleading, since we are not sure how we should describe the case of a patient with a terminal condition who "might easily avoid dying for a long time but might choose to end his life immediately by not taking cheap and painless medication" ([4], p. 86).

Beauchamp and Childress suggest the reason we have difficulty deciding the meaning of suicide is that the term has an emotive meaning of disapproval that we prefer not to apply to certain kinds of ambiguous cases. The very logic of the term therefore tends to prejudice any pending moral analysis of the rightness or wrongness of suicide. As a means to try to deal with this problem they propose an "uncorrupted" definition of suicide as what occurs "if and only if one intentionally terminates one's own life — no matter what the conditions or precise nature of the intention or the causal route to death" ([4], p. 87).[3]

As sympathetic as one must feel with their attempt to provide a clear and nonprejudicial account of suicide, however, the very idea of an "uncorrupted" definition of suicide distorts the very grammar of such notions. Beauchamp and Childress are quite right to point out that the notion itself cannot settle how and why suicide applies to certain kinds of behavior and not to others. But what must be admitted, as Joseph Margolis has argued, is the culturally variable character of suicide. There are many competing views about the meaning and nature of suicide,

> some religious, some not, some not even significantly so characterized. . . . There is no simple formula for designating, except trivially, an act of taking, or yielding, or making likely the end of, one's life that will count, universally, as suicide. No, some selection of acts of this minimal sort will, in accord with an interpreting tradition, construe what was done as or as not suicide; and so judging, the tradition will provide as well for the approval or condemnation of what was done. In short, suicide, like murder itself, is an act that can be specified only

in a systematic way within a given tradition; and that specification itself depends on classifying the intention of the agent. We can say, therefore, that there is no minimal act of commission or omission that counts as suicide, except relative to some tradition; and, within particular traditions, the justifiability of particular suicides may yet be debatable. ([13], p. 25-26)

So the very way one understands "suicide" already involves moral judgments and requires argument. I shall contend that if we rightly understand what life is about, suicide should be understood negatively and should not therefore be recommended as an alternative for anyone. This is not to deny that from certain perspectives suicide can be considered rational—as an institution, that is, a way of characterizing a whole range of behavior, as well as an individual act. That it can be so understood, however, reveals how little the issue turns on the question of "rationality." We must rather ask whether the tradition through which we understand the meaning and nature of suicide is true.

Why Suicide Is Prohibited

I have argued elsewhere that suicide as an institution must be considered morally doubtful. That conclusion is based on the religious understanding that we should learn to regard our lives as gifts bestowed on us by a gracious Creator ([11], pp. 101–115). That such an appeal is explicitly religious is undeniable, but I would resist any suggestion that the religious nature of this appeal disqualifies it from public argument. Rather it is a reminder of Margolis' contention that any account of suicide necessarily draws on some tradition. Therefore my appeal to this kind of religious presupposition is but an explicit avowal of what any account of suicide must involve—though I certainly would not contend that the only basis for disapproving suicide is religious.

It is important, however, that the significance of the shift to the language of gift be properly appreciated. For it is a challenge to our normal presumptions about the way the prohibition of suicide is grounded in our "natural desire to live." Indeed it is not even clear to me that we have a "natural desire to live," or even if we do what its moral significance entails. The very phrase "natural desire to live" is fraught with ambiguity, but, even worse, it seems to suggest that when a person no longer has such a desire there is no longer any reason for living.

In contrast, the language of gift does not presuppose we have a "natural desire to live," but rather that our living is an obligation. It is an obligation that we at once owe our Creator and one another. For our creaturely status is but a reminder that our existence is not secured by our own power, but rather requires the constant care of, and trust in, others. Our willingness to live in the face of suffering, pain, and sheer boredom of life is morally a service to one another as it is a sign that life can be endured and moreover our living can be done with joy and exuberance. Our obligation to sustain our lives even when they are threatened with, or require living with, a horrible disease is our way of being faithful to the trust that has sustained us in health and now in illness ([8], pp. 229–237). We take on a responsibility as sick people. That responsibility is simply to keep on living, as it is our way of gesturing to those who care for us that we can be trusted and trust them even in our illness.

There is nothing about this position which entails that we must do everything we can do to keep ourselves alive under all conditions. Christians certainly do not believe that life is inherently sacred and therefore it must be sustained until the bitter end. The existence of the martyrs is a clear sign that Christians think the value of life can be overridden [7]. Indeed I think there is much to be said for distinguishing between preserving life and only prolonging death, but such a distinction does not turn on technical judgments about when we have in fact started dying, though it may involve such a judgment ([12], pp. 166–186). Rather the distinction is dependent on the inherited wisdom of a community that has some idea of what a "good death" entails ([10], pp. 329–336).

Such a death is one that allows us to remember the dead in a morally healthy way — that is, the manner of death does not prevent the living from remembering the manner and good of their life. To be sure, we can train ourselves to remember a suicide as if the suicide said nothing about the life, but I think we would be unwise to do so. For to face the reality of a death by suicide is a reminder of how often our community fails to offer the trust necessary to sustain our lives in health and illness. Suicide is not first a judgment about the agent, but a reminder that we have failed to embody as a community the commitment not to abandon one another. We fear being a burden for others, but even more to ourselves. Yet it is only by recognizing that in fact we are inescapably a burden that we face the reality and opportunity of living truthfully.

It is just such a commitment that medicine involves and this is why the physician's commitment to caring for the sick seems so distorted by an ethics of autonomy. Medicine is but a gesture, but an extremely significant gesture of a society, that while we all suffer from a condition that cannot be cured, nonetheless neither will we be abandoned. The task of medicine is to care even when it cannot cure ([11], pp. 145–150). The refusal to let an attempted suicide die is only our feeble, but real, attempt to remain a community of trust and care through the agency of medicine. Our prohibition and subsequent care of a suicide draws on our profoundest assumptions that each individual's life has a purpose beyond simply being "autonomous."

Reasons for Living and "Rational Suicide": An Example

However, the kind of religious appeal I have made as well as this kind of talk about "purpose" can easily be misleading. For it sounds as though suicide is religiously prohibited because people who believe in God really know what life is about. But that is not the case — at least in the usual sense that the phrase "what life is about" is understood. Indeed the very reason that living is an obligation is that we are to go on living even though we are far from figuring out what life is about. Our reason for living is not that we are sure about the ultimate meaning of life, but rather because our lives have been touched by another and through that touch we believe we encounter the very being that graciously sustains our existence.

Indeed one of the problems with discussions of "rational suicide" is that they seem to be determined by the assumption that the decision to live or to die turns on whether life, and more importantly, one's particular life, has meaning or purpose. Thus, Margolis, for example, suggests that the question raised by a relatively neutral understanding of suicide is whether the deliberate taking of one's life in order simply to end it, not instrumentally for any ulterior purpose, can ever be rational or rationally justified. He suggests a rational suicide is a person who "aims overridingly at ending his own life and who, in a relevant sense, performs the act. The manner in which he suicides may be said to be by commission or omission, actively or passively, directly or indirectly, consciously or unconsciously, justifiably or reprehensibly — in accord with the classificatory distinctions of particular traditions" ([13], p. 29). According to Margolis, such suicide is more likely to be justified if the person "decided that life was utterly meaningless or sincerely believed life to have no point at all" ([13], p. 24).

My difficulty with such a suggestion is that I have no idea what it would mean to know that life, and particularly my life, was "utterly meaningless" or had "no point at all." In order to illustrate my difficulty about these matters let me call your attention to one of the better books about suicide — John Barth's *The Floating Opera*.[4] Barth's book consists of Todd Andrews' account of how one day in 1937 he decided to commit suicide. There was no particular reason that Andrews decided to commit suicide and that, we discover, is exactly the reason he decided to do so — namely there is no reason for living or dying.

The protagonist has written the book to explain why he changed his mind and in the process we discover quite a bit about him. Most people would describe him as a cynic, but there is more to him than that. Andrews makes his living by practicing law in a small backwater town in the Chesapeake tidewater country. He became a lawyer because that is what his father wanted, but he is later stunned by his father's suicide. What bothered him was not that his father killed himself, but that he did so because he could not pay his debts due to the depression.

Andrews has chosen to live free from any long-term commitments since the day in World War I when he killed a German sergeant with whom he had shared a foxhole through a terrible night of shelling. His lack of commitment extends even to his arrangement for living — he lives in a hotel room where he registers on a day-to-day basis. He has, however, been involved in a long-term affair with Jane Mack, his best friend's wife. Harrison Mack not only approved but actually arranged this as a further extension of their friendship. However by mutual agreement they have recently decided to end this form of their relationship.[5] This is partly the result of the recent birth of Jeannie, who, even though her paternity remains unclear, has given the Macks a new sense of themselves as a couple.

Andrews also suffers from two diseases — subacute bacteriological endocarditis and chronic infection of the prostate. He was told thirty-five years ago that the former could kill him any time. The latter disease only caused him to cease living the wastrel's existence he had assumed during law school and begin what he claims is almost a saintly life. And indeed his life is in many way exemplary, for he is a man who lives his life in accordance with those convictions he thinks most nearly true.

Even though he is not a professional philosopher, Andrews is a person with a definite philosophical bent. For years he has been working on notes, suitably filed in three peach baskets, for the writing of a Humean type *Inquiry* on the nature of causation. For if Hume was right that causes can only be inferred, then his task is to shorten as much as possible the leap between what we see to what we cannot see — that is, to get at the true reasons for our actions.[6]

This becomes particularly relevant if we are to understand Andrews' decision to commit suicide. He fully admits that there are abundant psychological reasons, for those inclined for such explanations, to explain his suicide — a motherless boyhood, his murder of the German sergeant, his father's hanging himself, his isolated adulthood, his ailing heart, his growing sexual impotency, injured vanity, frustrated ambition, boredom — the kinds of things psychoanalysts identify as "real" causes ([2], p. 224). But for him the only reasons that interest him in dying are philosophical, which he states in five propositions which constitute his completed *Inquiry*. They simply are:

I. Nothing has intrinsic value. Things assume value only in terms of certain ends.

II. The reasons for which people attribute value to things are always ultimately arbitrary. That is, the ends in terms of which things assume value are themselves ultimately irrational.

III. There is, therefore, no ultimate 'reason' for valuing anything.

IV. Living is action in some form. There is no reason for action in any form.

V. There is, then, no 'reason' for living. ([2], pp. 238-243)

And so Todd Andrews made up his mind to kill himself one day in 1937.

However before doing so he decided to go see *The Original and Unparalleled Floating Opera*, a local minstrel show on a run-down showboat. The absurdity of the show matches perfectly Andrews' view of the absurdity of life. During the performance, Andrews goes to the ship's galley, turns on the gas, only to be interrupted and saved by a workman who angrily calls him a damn fool — not because he tried to take his life, but because he could have blown up the ship.

More importantly, however, just as he is recovering, the Macks, who had also been attending the *Opera*, rush into the galley with Jeannie, who has suddenly taken sick and fainted. Though appealed to for help, Andrews suggests he is not good at such things and advises the Macks to go to the hospital. However, the local doctor arrives and advises an alcohol rub, reassuring everyone nothing is seriously wrong. In the emergency and the concern Andrews felt about Jeannie, he discovers he no longer wants to commit suicide, even though he could still easily jump into the Choptank River. For, as he tells us,

> Something was different. Some qualitative change had occurred, instantly, down in the dining room. The fact is I had no reason to be concerned over little Jeannie, and yet my concern for that child was so intense, and had been so immediately forthcoming, that (I understood now) the first desperate sound of Jane's voice had snapped me out of a paralysis which there was no reason to terminate. No reason at all. Moreover, had I not, in abjuring my responsibility for Jeannie, for the first time in my life assumed it—for her, for her parents, and for myself? I was confused, and I refused to die that way. Things needed explaining; abstractions needed to be straightened out. To die now was simply out of the question, though I hated to spoil such a perfect day. ([2], p. 266)

Andrews suspects most philosophizing to be rationalization but nonetheless his experience requires him to return to the propositions of his *Inquiry* to make a small revision of the fifth: "V. There is, then, no 'reason' for living (or for suicide)" ([2]:270). For now he tells us that he realized that even if values are only relative there are still relative values.

> To realize that nothing has absolute value is, surely, overwhelming, but if one goes no further from that proposition than to become a saint, a cynic, or a suicide on principle, one hasn't gone far enough. If nothing makes any final difference, that fact makes no final difference either, and there is no more reason to commit suicide, say, than not to, in the last analysis. Hamlet's question is, absolutely, meaningless. A narrow escape. ([2], p. 270)

The Christian prohibition of suicide is clearly based in our assumption that our lives are not ours to do with as we please. But that prohibition is but a reminder of the kind of commitments that make suicide, which appears from certain perspectives and at particular times in our lives so rational, so wrong. It reminds us of our commitment to be the kind of people who can care about a sick little girl and in the process we learn to care for ourselves. That kind of lesson may not give life meaning, but it is certainly sufficient to help us muddle through with enough joy to sustain the important business of living.

NOTES

1. For example Beauchamp and Childress ([4], p. 90) suggest, "If the principle of autonomy is strongly relied upon for the justification of suicide, then it would seem that there is a right to commit suicide, so long as a person acts autonomously and does not seriously affect the interests of others." Beauchamp and Childress continue to maintain this position in the second edition of their book. In particular see p. 99 of second edition (1983).

2. Earlier Augustine had argued, "There were famous heroes who, though by the laws of war they could do violence to a conquered enemy, refuse to do violence to themselves when conquered; though they had not the slightest fear of death, they chose to endure the enemy's domination rather than put themselves to death. They were fighting for their earthly country; but the Gods they worshipped were false; but their worship was genuine and they faithfully kept their oaths. Christians worship the true God and they yearn for a heavenly country; will they not have more reason to refrain from the crime of suicide, if God's providence subjects them for a time to their enemies for their probation or reformation. Their God does not abandon them in that humiliation, for he came from on high so humbly for their sake" ([1], pp. 35-36).

3. In the second edition of their book Beauchamp and Childress note that their more "objective" definition of suicide is nonetheless "stipulative" (1983, p. 94). Elsewhere Beauchamp provides a fuller account, arguing suicide occurs when "a person intentionally brings about his or her own death in circumstances where others do not coerce him or her in the action, except in those cases where death is caused by conditions not specifically arranged by the agent for the purpose of bringing about his or her own death" ([3], p. 77).

4. For a similar approach from which I have learned much see Nielsen [14]. The fact that we must resort to example when considering such matters is an important indication of how abstract discussions of the rightness or wrongness of suicide, for which there is no substitute and must certainly be

done, can as easily mislead as they can help us clarify why the suicide is rightly understood in a negative manner. Seldom are any of us sure why it is we act and do not act as we do. We may say we would rather die than live with such and such disease, but how can we be so sure that is the reason. Beauchamp and Childress' suggestion that ideally a person contemplating suicide would consider all the variables is as much a formula for self-deception as one for self-knowledge. I suspect that is why Barth's book is so helpful — namely, it is only by telling a story that we come to understand how the prohibition against suicide is meant to shape the self.

5. Andrews admits that this turn of affairs made him reconsider briefly his decision to commit suicide, since the Macks might interpret his suicide as caused by their decision. But he says that this lasted only a moment, since it occurred to him "What difference did it make to me how they interpreted my death? Nothing, absolutely, makes any difference. Nothing is ultimately important. And that, at least partly by my own choosing, that last act would be robbed of its real significance, would be interpreted in every way but the way I intended. This fact once realized, it seemed likely to me that here was a new significance, if possible even more genuine" ([2], p. 224).

6. The full title is actually *On Inquiry into the Circumstances Surrounding the Self-Destruction of Thomas Andrews, of Cambridge, Maryland, on Ground-Hog Day, 1930 (More Especially into the Causes Therefor)*. For Andrews tells us his aim is simply to learn why his father hanged himself. Andrews admits the real problem was one of "imperfect communication" between him and his father, as he could find no adequate reason for his father's act. His *Inquiry*, however, became primarily a study of himself, since he realized that to understand imperfect communications requires perfect knowledge of each party. Andrews suggests at the end of the book that if we have not understood his change of mind he is again cursed with imperfect communication — but the suggestion seems to be that we have a better chance at communication than he had with his father, as now at least we have Todd Andrews' story.

REFERENCES

[1] Augustine. 1977. *The City of God*. Trans. Henry Bettenson. Harmondsworth: Penguin.
[2] Barth, J. 1956. *The Floating Opera*. New York: Avon.
[3] Beauchamp, T. 1980. "Suicide." In T. Regan, ed., *Matters of Life and Death*, 67–108. New York: Random House.
[4] Beauchamp, T., and Childress, J. 1979. *Principles of Biomedical Ethics*. New York: Oxford University Press.

[5] Bergmann, F. 1977. *On Being Free*. Notre Dame, Ind.: University of Notre Dame Press.

[6] Dworkin, G. 1978. "Moral Autonomy." In H. Engelhardt and D. Callahan, eds., *Morals, Science and Sociality*, 156–171. Hastings-on-Hudson, N.Y.: Hastings Center Publication.

[7] Hauerwas, S. 1980. *Community of Character*. Notre Dame, Ind.: University of Notre Dame Press.

[8] Hauerwas, S. 1979. "Reflections on Suffering, Death, and Medicine." *Ethics in Science and Medicine* 6: 229–237. Reprinted in the present volume (See essay no. 1).

[9] Hauerwas, S. 1978. "Care." In W. Reich, ed., *Encyclopedia of Bioethics*, 145–150. New York: Free Press.

[10] Hauerwas, S. 1978a."Religious Concepts of Brain Death." *New York Academy of Sciences Annals* 215: 329–338. Reprinted in the present volume (See essay no. 4).

[11] Hauerwas, S. 1977. *Truthfulness and Tragedy*. Notre Dame, Ind.: University of Notre Dame Press.

[12] Hauerwas, S. 1974. *Vision and Virtue*. Notre Dame, Ind.: Fides Claretian; rpt. University of Notre Dame Press, 1981.

[13] Margolis, J. 1975. *Negativities: The Limits of Life*. Columbus, Ohio: Merrill.

[14] Nielsen, H. 1979. "Margolis on Rational Suicide: An Argument for Case Studies in Ethics." *Ethics* 89, no. 4: 394–400.

6

Ethical Issues in the Use
of Human Subjects

The Variety of Ethical Analysis

The ethical issues surrounding human experimentation are complex and, I suspect, some of them are irresolvable in a society like ours. I am going to try to describe how ethicists tend to frame the ethical concerns involved in the experimental use of human subjects. However, I must ask you to keep in mind that there is no ethically neutral way to describe a moral problem. Indeed the very designation of a "problem" depends on prior moral presuppositions. For example, different positions concerning the use of human subjects are often thought to be determined by whether a deontological or teleological pattern of moral justifications is dominant. Yet this very way of construing the dispute may conceal a more fundamental disagreement about how to describe morally what human experimentation involves. Thus while I am trying to act primarily as a reporter, you should suspect that my commitments color the way I describe the ethical issues involved in the use of human subjects in research.

Protection of the Individual Versus the Benefit to Humankind

Perhaps the most basic as well as the most heated issue surrounding the use of human subjects in research is the assumption by some that the primary ethical question is whether the benefits of any research are sufficient to justify certain risks to the subject. In other words many in the research community seem to assume that the question of the moral justification of research on human beings is a matter of providing more information about comparative benefits and risks. The experiment is thought justified if it has been carefully designed and can be shown that the actual or potential benefit outweighs the risk.

114

Others, however, have argued that this way of stating the moral issue is to beg the principal moral question. They argue that the teleological assumption — that is, the idea that the good consequences outweigh the bad — involved in this kind of ethical cost-benefit analysis fails to do justice to the basic commitment to respect and protect each human person. Put differently, it is argued that no amount of benefit can ever justify using one person as a means for the good of others. Those who assume that the ethical issue is one of balancing some risks against future goods fail to see, therefore, that respect for the integrity of the individual cannot be balanced by the benefits gained — no matter how the benefits might be understood. Thus Jay Katz argues that what must be recognized is that there is an inherent value conflict in the conduct of human research — "the quest for the acquisition of knowledge for the benefit of present and future generations on the one hand; and the respect for the dignity, autonomy, and inviolability (unless consented to) of the subjects of research" ([4], p. 154).

Those who argue that the protection of the human subject is the overriding ethical issue for human experimentation do not intend this demand to deny any use of human subjects in research. Rather they argue that any experiment must provide proper safeguards for the human subject. If such safeguards cannot be provided, then the experiment cannot be done even if it would have great benefit for present and future generations. Ethically this means that no basic value can be overridden for a higher good, except if it can be shown that another basic value is at stake. Many scientists find such a position unduly restrictive as they cannot understand why the attempt to eliminate disease is not a "basic good" that justifies the use of some for that good.

If the Conference on Experiments and Research with Humans sponsored by the National Academy of Sciences in 1975[1] was any example, I am afraid that we have a long way to go before this conflict is resolved. (Moreover, it is hard to see how we can expect it to be solved at the policy level when it has not been resolved at the level of ethical theory.) For neither side seems to be able to speak to the concerns of the other. Scientists cannot understand how anyone can fail to appreciate the benefits to be gained through science for the good of mankind. Talk of the "inviolability of the individual" appears as an irrational commitment that is holding back important developments for the cure of disease or opening up new vistas of human understanding.

Those concerned with the protection of human subjects as the overriding value, however, tend to think that research scientists naively assume that what is good for science is also good for mankind. Just as what is good for business is not necessarily good for America, they argue that the assumed importance of science for human betterment, both morally and materially, must be shown rather than simply asserted. For scientists often seem to assume that their activity can be justified on the simple utilitarian grounds of the greatest good for the greatest number. Yet utilitarianism as an ethical theory remains problematic because it fails to account for some of our central intuitions about what we can justly do and not do.

Even though I am sympathetic with those who have argued for the priority of protection of the human subject, I think they have not as yet provided convincing grounds for their allegiance to the individual. Ramsey's contention that "no man is good enough to experiment upon another without his consent" ([6], p. 59), seems to strike a chord within us, but it is not clear why this is the case. Of course it is possible to argue within the framework of liberal political theory that we simply have a "right" not to be subjected to the interests of others. This response continues to assume that we have a clear idea of what "rights" involve or how they can be justified. But this is not the case.

As Alasdair MacIntyre has recently observed,

It is an interesting paradox that those eighteenth century writers such as Jefferson or Robespierre who believed they intuited timeless truths about the rights of man did so in a vocabulary that had historically come into existence as a child of late medieval legal usage and which does not seem to be found in the precise senses in which they used it until a hundred and fifty years or so before their own time. But it is easy to understand why it did emerge as a central moral as well as legal concept. The central preoccupation of both ancient and medieval communities was characteristically: how may men together realize the true human good? The central preoccupation of modern men is and has been characteristically: how may we prevent men interfering with each other as each of us goes about our own concerns? The classical view begins with the community of the *polis* and with the individual viewed as having no moral identity apart from the communities of kinship and citizenship; the modern view begins with the concept of a collection of individuals and the problem of how out of and by individuals social institutions can be constructed. ([5], Essay 10, pp. 22-23)

If MacIntyre is right about this, and I think he is, then in an interesting way the appeal to "rights" to protect research subjects presupposes the same individualistic presuppositions as utilitarianism. This may reveal that, while appearing antagonistic, the teleologist and deontologist on this issue may actually share some of the same presuppositions. Or, more accurately, it helps us to see that to construe the issue of the use of human subjects in terms of a choice between teleological or deontological ethical theories is misleading. For the issue is what kind of risks we as citizens and recipients of the benefits of health science should be willing to undergo to further the general well-being of our community.

But if this is the right way to frame the question, it cannot be answered in terms of the current discussion, but must await the development of a new sense of political community and resulting political and ethical theory. For only then can we stand back from abstractions such as "the good of mankind" or "the rights of the individual" and be clear about what ends and values science can and should serve. With the articulation of such ends we may well find the grounds to say why each of us should be willing to serve as research subjects for the good, not of mankind, but of the communities in which we exist.[2] Because we do not share these values, however, the only way we feel that we can protect ourselves from one another is by insisting on the procedural rule of informed consent. In other words, what we have here is the typical liberal strategy to substitute procedure where debate on substantive norms and values is lacking.

Therapeutic and Nontherapeutic Experimentation

It can be objected that I have overstated the unclarity of the moral values and ends that give direction to contemporary research. To be sure, there is an important distinction between therapeutic and nontherapeutic experimentation that suggests we have a clearer idea of what we are doing in therapeutic cases. But we also know that this distinction is often easier to draw in theory than it is in practice. For example, there are good grounds to think, in spite of the wide practice of kidney transplants, that such a procedure is still an experimental technique ([1], pp. 60-108). Furthermore, it remains unclear if random clinical trials should be viewed as therapeutic or nontherapeutic, even though medical progress depends on such testing.[3] For the issue is: medical progress for whom — the immediately sick person or future patient populations?

The question of who the doctor's patient is or should be is often not easy to determine, but it is complicated by the realization that we are no longer sure what health and illness mean. As Charles Fried has suggested, "The concept of good health implies a concept of the good life, and the goodness of life includes a large number of other factors besides simply its length" ([2], p. 50). Thus the doctor's primary duty is not the prevention of death, but rather the preservation of bodily integrity necessary for the realization of a reasonable and realistic life plan ([3], pp. 11-42).[4] But we have little consensus about what kind of medicine should be developed because we are unclear what constitutes a "reasonable and realistic life plan." Concretely this means we have no way of determining whether we should develop heart transplant procedures in order to provide some with opportunities not normally thought to be a possibility. Moreover we are increasingly seeing the development of such procedures result in a two-tiered medical system — it's one for those who can pay and another for those who are "uninsured."

Even if we knew better what health means or should mean it is unclear how this would help us direct the research not directly associated with therapeutic ends. For example, some of the hard cases involving the use of human subjects in research are clearly nontherapeutic — that is, the research aims to obtain information of use to others and thus does not pretend to treat some illness that the experimental subject might have. Thus the need for justification for using human subjects in such research is made more intense because the design and ends of such experiments are remote from the therapeutic context.

Informed Consent

Of course many assume that the requirement of "informed consent" is a sufficient safeguard to protect subjects involved in therapeutic and nontherapeutic experimentation. Informed consent at least means that the doctor or the experimenter must give the subject the facts necessary to make an informed choice. That means that if the subject is ill he must have a clear sense of the diagnosis of his illness and the prognosis without treatment. Also the patient must have an idea of the benefits and risks of the treatment as well as the hazards and advantages of alternative forms of treatment.

Fried summarizes the rules that define informed consent as: "1) A fair explanation of the procedures to be followed, and their purpose, including identification of any procedures which are experimental; 2) A description of the attendant discomforts and risks reasonably to be expected; 3) A description of any benefits reasonably to be expected; 4) A disclosure of any appropriate alternative procedures that might be advantageous for the subject; 5) An offer to answer any inquiries concerning the procedures; and 6) An instruction that the subject is free to withdraw his consent and to discontinue participation in the project activity at any time" ([2], p. 42).

As it stands, this sounds fine, and it surely acts as a brake on some of the abuses that might occur if we did not require it. The problem, however, with informed consent being used as the overriding justification criterion for experimentation is that few believe it is really possible to obtain. For many doctors, informed consent is that slip of paper that is a necessary (but as we have discovered, not sufficient) condition to avoid malpractice. But even if the doctor or researcher is committed to informed consent it is not clear that it describes a genuine choice. As a famous heart surgeon once told me, for a patient to make an informed decision to undergo heart surgery would mean he would have to study with him for at least three years (and that was assuming the patient had completed medical school). Though this certainly overstates the case, one may still ask whether informed consent is workable in practice.

Even if informed consent were a clear possibility, it is still not a sufficient condition to justify human experimentation. In some form or other, informed consent is probably a necessary condition for the use of human subjects, but simply because some may consent to make themselves subject to an experiment does not mean that they should so consent. For persons can misuse themselves even if they do so voluntarily and with full knowledge. There are some things that we should not do to ourselves even for the good of others. To absolutize informed consent does not resolve the issue of whether we ought to allow ourselves to be subjected to certain kinds of risks in the name of human good.

Nor is this kind of problem limited to those experiments which involve the greater physical risk to the subject. Indeed, I think that the issue is even more important in relation to the kind of experiments in the social and psychological sciences where deception is necessary to the experimental design. It is important to remember that we can morally harm without physically hurting.

Even if we can make informed consent a workable criterion for human experimentation there remains the problem of what we do about particular test populations. Should prisoners or the poor be subjected to human experimentation? Many argue that because of their disadvantaged position any informed consent they might give, in spite of elaborate safeguards, is inherently coercive. However, Katz suggests that this attitude, especially toward the poor, betrays a stereotypical and degrading view of them ([4], p. 154). To be sure, it may be necessary to exercise special care in respect to prisoners and the poor, but to deny them the opportunity to participate in the joint venture of our community to better our condition is to deny them the respect due them. (The situation of the poor may be significantly different than that of prisoners, however, insofar as the latter have no power to protect themselves. This may also be important in the use of students in research, for while they appear free, they are in fact in a disadvantaged position since their future depends on being able to please professors. At the very least, this means that the manner of obtaining informed consent is very important in contexts where the one consenting lacks the power to withstand the suggestion that he volunteer. This is especially the case when the "power" is unarticulated and informal.)

Of course, for this last point to be viable depends on the actual existence of that joint venture. Yet, in fact, we know that doctors and medical researchers have gone to great lengths to avoid exposing the general population to the risks necessary for medical advances. This is not the place to speculate about the reasons for this, though I suspect it has much to do with the paternalistic attempt of doctors to protect us from the risks involved in normal medicine, but until medical experimentation is seen as an opportunity—and perhaps even an obligation—for everyone, I find it hard to justify the continued use of prisoners and the poor as experimental subjects. Moreover, if we were willing to widen the opportunity for more people to participate in scientific research, it would necessitate the healthy development of making the scientific community take the time to explain what they are about.

Or put more positively, it would help us see the stake we all have, and the risk we should assume, for the development of certain kinds of research.

The ethical issues raised by the use of prisoners and the poor seem simple when compared to the problems involved in the use of children and other non-competents. In order to develop certain kinds of drugs or procedures we can do all the animal and adult testing we want and still we must finally test on children—i.e., a test group who by definition cannot give informed consent. Paul Ramsey has argued that no one, parent or guardian, even with the best intentions, has the moral status to give consent for a child to be made the subject of medical investigation solely for the accumulation of knowledge (except when epidemic conditions prevail). To quote: "When there is no possible relation to the child's recovery, a child is not to be made a mere object in medical experimentation for the good to come" ([6], p. 12). If it is objected that this severely restricts possible advances in childhood medicine, Ramsey argues that the moral progress of the race is more important than the scientific. Thus, testing on children is the paradigm instance that at times it may be necessary to choose between morality and knowledge even though we normally assume that we do not have to choose between them.

(Without developing it I at least want to suggest that not enough attention has been paid to the ethical issues involved in using animals in research. It may well be that we will learn more about what moral issues are involved in human research if we think more about our assumption that we can subject animals to almost any peril or pain for the good of people. Our inhumanity to our fellow man may well be a correlative to our unjustified insensitivity to those not of our species.)

The Basis of Informed Consent

In conclusion I think it is interesting to ask why we have come to think that informed consent is so important. Above I have quoted Ramsey to the effect that no man is good enough to experiment upon another without his consent, but it is not clear why this is the case. Of course many would argue that no man has the right to force another to do what he does not want to, even if it will have positive benefits for others. In the framework of the libertarian political ethic this response has some plausibility, but as I suggested, this involves an individualist assumption that avoids asking what ends medicines and collateral research ought to serve.

In this connection Charles Fried's recent analysis of the basis of informed consent seems to me to be particularly suggestive and illuminating ([2], pp. 67-68). Fried argues that our commitment to the individual subject is based on the idea that the ethical life is primarily anchored in the concrete relationships in which we are involved. In other words, Fried suggests that the sense of care we should have for others is not based on impersonal moral principles, but grows out of our more or less direct commitment to particular significant others. Thus we feel that we have obligations to our wives, children, and friends which are qualitatively different from obligations to those with whom we are not in such relationship. Moreover, we feel that whatever our obligations to a stranger may be, they cannot override our obligation to those with whom we share a special relationship. If Fried is right, our obligation to the stranger is based on our prior commitment to particular friendships.

Fried goes on to argue that the kind of relationship between a doctor and his patient is of this primary sort. Thus the ethos of medicine assures the patient that the doctor's concern for him or her is absolute — that is, it would be immoral for the doctor ever to lower the quality of care of one patient for the good of another even if the "another" were a greater number. The requirement of informed and free consent for therapeutic as well as experimental procedures refers to one attempt to safeguard our fundamental commitment, then, to primary relationships. It is to be noted therefore that the concern with the "rights" of the human subject is not necessarily based on the inviolability of the individual, but rather grounded on the community possible between those who wish to be friends.

But if Fried has properly identified the relationship which underwrites the doctor's sense of commitment to each individual patient, it must be asked how this commitment translates into the nontherapeutic experimental context? If this is not the kind of relationship between the scientist and the human subject, then even more careful procedure must be developed in the research context to protect the subject. For we must see that what we have is not a joint venture for medical progress or human goods secured through such progress, but a relationship between strangers in which one side has been given more power than the other in the name of science.

NOTES

1. For the proceedings of this conference see (4).

2. Fox and Swazey put this well as they suggest that "the social and cultural meaning of dialysis and transplantation is also integral to the question these procedures have raised about the basis and significance of human solidarity. The nature and importance of our relationship to one another is a core issue in every society, system of ethics, and religion. Dialysis and transplantation have reemphasized how central it is to medicine as well. This has occurred in a period of generalized crisis even whether and how an advantaged society like our own can achieve a more trusting intimate, inclusive, and transcendent form of solidarity" ([1], p. 330–331).

3. Charles Fried, ([2]). Randomized clinical trial is the therapeutic investigation "in which the allocation of a patient to a particular treatment category or its alternative—sometimes an alternative therapy, sometimes a placebo, that is no therapy at all—is done at random," ([2], p. 7). Of course part of the problem with this procedure is that the patient is drafted into it without his or her knowledge, since part of the value of the trial depends on the patient not knowing other therapeutic alternatives are available. It is assumed that this is justified because in such an experiment no technique has shown itself to be superior to another.

4. I am obviously sympathetic to Kass's general perspective, though I am not as confident as he that we can develop an ontologically compelling account of the "organism as a whole" by which we can determine the meaning of health.

REFERENCES

[1] Fox, Renee, and Swazey, Judith. 1974. *The Courage to Fail*. Chicago: University of Chicago Press.
[2] Fried, Charles. 1974. *Medical Experimentation: Personal Integrity and Social Policy*. New York: American Elsevier Publishing Co.
[3] Kass, Leon. 1975 "Regarding the End of Medicine and the Pursuit of Health," *The Public Interest* 40: 11-12. This essay has recently been

reprinted in Leon Kass, *Toward a More Natural Science*. New York: Free Press, pp. 157–186.

[4] Katz, Jay. 1975. "The Poor." In *Experiments and Research with Humans: Values in Conflict*. Washington, D.C.: National Academy of Science.

[5] MacIntyre, Alasdair. 1982. "How to Identify Ethical Principles." In *The Belmont Report*, DHEW Publication, No. (OS) 78-0013, Washington, D.C.

[6] Ramsey, Paul. 1970. *The Patient as Person*. New Haven: Yale University Press.

7

Rights, Duties, and Experimentation on Children

Do Children Have or Need "Rights"?

When confronted by questions of how to approach research on children we seem drawn to the language of rights. Rights seem to offer the kind of protection we think children should have. Yet I think it is extremely doubtful if rights are appropriately attributed to children (or anyone else for that matter). It will be the primary burden of this essay[1] to suggest why such is the case. As an alternative to rights language I will try to show why the language of duties is more to the point.

That "rights" are thought to be the primary question when confronted with issues raised by experimentation on children is but a manifestation of how liberal societies tend to substitute procedural requirements for substantive judgments. Since it is the hallmark of liberal societies to allow each man and woman to marry for any reason and to have children for any reason, then it makes little sense for such a society to try to include a normative conception of family and parental responsibility in its national policies. To employ the language of rights is to assume that children are simply one interest group among others and that they must have procedural safeguards in order to be protected from the undue advantage of other interest groups, including their parents.

The requirement of parental consent for medical treatment of a child was originally based on the assumption that the parents were those who knew and cared the most about the interests of the child. To be sure, this assumption opened the way for unwarranted interference or, conversely, noninvolvement by parents, but there was a check on parental misjudgment as well as malicious intent. That check was a normative view of the family that was widely shared by the surrounding community — a view which included patterns of parental responsibility and expectations concerning how one ought to care for children.

The employment of the language of rights is an attempt to make up for the breakdown of our shared beliefs about how parents should care for their children. In such a context parental consent is seen not as a safeguard in respect to powers the child would not otherwise know how to handle but as an unwarranted and arbitrary power of parents over children. The use of the language of rights in relation to children appears, then, to be a moral advance, since such putative "rights" seem to give the child standing over against the parents as well as society.

However in our enthusiasm for the renewed appreciation of the standing of children that "rights" language seems to entail, we may have avoided entirely the issue of what kind of responsibilities parents should have toward their children. To answer that question involves knowing why people should have children at all, what level of care parents should be able to provide for the nourishing of children, and to what sacrifices and risks children should be exposed.

(The problem of exposing our children to risks is tied to our difficulty of knowing when it is appropriate to let children die. Indeed I suspect some of the worst cruelty perpetrated on children today results not from malicious intent, but from parental fear. Confused about what we should do when our children are threatened with death, we are tempted to do too much lest we not do enough. The urgency behind some forms of research on children derives, I think, from an unwarranted desire to keep our children alive beyond all reason. Death is never pleasant, nor is it anything that any of us should want, but there comes a time to die, even for children.)

Of course there is another way to interpret the use of rights language in terms of research on children. To claim "rights" for the family can be thought equivalent to claiming that the state has no competency in matters dealing with the family; that freedom means that the state cannot and should not interfere with how families are formed and children raised. However this sense of "rights" is not germane to our case, because in this sense the subject of the "rights" is not the child but the family unit itself.

Moreover this sense of "the family's rights" cannot be maintained without qualification, even in a liberal state. The state does have a stake in how families are formed and children cared for, even if it is in a minimalistic sense. Parents cannot subject their children to cruel or inhumane treatment. Parents are expected to provide their children basic forms of medical care in order to protect them from serious infectious diseases. Moreover, parents are obligated to educate their children in a manner appropriate to the parent's basic convictions. That these expectations be met is important to the continued functioning of the state.

The question of the use of children as subjects of experimental research is but one further activity in which the state has a responsibility toward children. This is especially the case when most of that research is directly or indirectly sponsored by the state through grants or agency involvement. It is not a question of whether the state is or is not involved with the family in these cases, but rather *how* the state should be involved and what conception of children and parental responsibility toward children should guide the state's policy. It is simply not possible for the state to act as if it can take a neutral stance toward the kind of responsibility parents have for their children. The language of the rights of children may appear to be less controversial, since it lets the state appear to be interfering less in how individual families are formed, but in fact it embodies a normative conception of the family that may be destructive of parental responsibility to care for and protect their children.

The Ethical Presuppositions of the Appeal to Rights

Rights language, however, appears to be a powerful idiom for consideration of these issues not only because of its social context, but because it is the language most natural to contemporary ethical theory. Most ethical theory since Kant has tried to base moral obligation on as thin a view of human nature and relations as possible. What we owe one another, it is thought, should be based not on being a father, citizen, or teacher but on our capacity for rational thought. The language of rights is a natural language for such a theory, since morally, rights are those claims that can be made irrespective of any special, historical, or personal relations in which we may find ourselves.

Put differently, contemporary ethical theory has avoided dealing with issues such as the nature of the family exactly because its presuppositions make the family appear odd or at least not an ethically interesting object for analysis. For we need to remember the language of rights is of recent origin and presupposes an individualistic understanding of the person in society. Rights are necessary when it is assumed that citizens fundamentally relate to one another as strangers, if not outright enemies. From such a perspective society appears as a collection of individuals who of necessity must enter into a bargain to insure their individual survival through providing for the survival of the society.

This conception of society makes it appear that all social relations in one way or another take the form of a contract through which all human relations are commercialized. The use of rights language in relation to the family, therefore, yields an understanding of the family as a contractual society of individuals. But that is exactly what it is not. In the language of Aristotle, the family is a "natural" institution. "Nature" does not mean that it is clear that we must form families in order to satisfy basic desires, but rather the family is a primitive institution prior to that of the state. We do not ask to be born into families, we simply *are* born into families of one kind or another. In a decisive sense the family is not a voluntary institution and the kind of responsibilities that accrue in it are thus different.

Moreover, because of its peculiar interest in freeing ethical judgments from all contingent beliefs and practices, contemporary ethical theory has failed to pay sufficient attention to the kind of moral role that is implied by the notion of "child." It has simply assumed that we know what we mean morally when we speak of children — namely, those who are smaller, younger, dependent, and less "rational" than adults. But if the argument above has been correct we cannot know what it means to be a child unless we have some normative understanding of what it means to be a family. "Child" and "children" denote moral roles that are relative to a set of expectations and practices that we call family.

It is certainly true that the moral meaning of being a child has changed through history and differed from one society to another. But that simply reinforces the point that morally the notion of family and child is dependent on a moral and historical development our society has inherited and changed. I am suggesting that basic to that history was the assumption that parents had duties toward the child not simply because they were responsible for bringing the child into existence, but because being a parent involved performing an office for the community to see that the child was cared for and educated in a manner appropriate to that community.

Perhaps the point I am trying to make can be best illustrated by calling attention to the place of the family in some of the more conservative religious traditions. For the Orthodox Jew there is no question of whether he or she should or should not have a family; children are a religious duty for the continuation of the people of Israel. To be a parent in such a context means that you have duties to fulfill; you must care for children in a manner appropriate to making them full participants in your community. That may not mean giving them all the medical care available; learning the Torah may in fact be more important. As a parent you do not impose your will on the child in an arbitrary manner; rather you act as an officer of the community to initiate the child into the practices of that community. The child does not have "rights" *qua* human being, but the child does have a standing as an independent agent in relation to its parents because both parents and child are subject to the community's expectations. Morally, the meaning of "child" is relative to the interests and needs of the community as mediated through the family. You are no longer a child when you can observe the Torah.

I am not trying to defend any one view of the family by appealing to this example; rather I am trying to make the conceptual point that any appeal to family or child as moral entities requires a set of historical presuppositions. In other words, to speak of family and child is exactly to speak of the duties of parents and children toward one another that are grounded in the concrete expectations of particular communities. But it has been the pretension of modern ethical theory that it could free itself from such historical presuppositions and ground moral judgments in man's "rational" nature *qua* man—i.e., as if we were strangers to one another in the sense that we share no history or common purposes. That is to isolate the family from any context in which it morally can make sense.

In summary, modern ethical theory has tried to deal with the issues of the status of children as research subjects in the language of rights because such language best suits its own methodological commitments. The language of rights appears to provide a way of giving children a moral status without presupposing any arbitrary and particular conception of parental responsibility. However, I have tried to suggest that even though such a strategy may have some plausibility in a society where parental responsibility is unclear and ambiguous, the strategy in fact embodies assumptions that contribute to the distortion of the family as a moral entity.

The Cogency of Rights Language

My argument is not meant to deny all cogency to rights language, but rather to suggest that appeal to rights cannot provide the kind of basic moral presuppositions needed for the social and political life of a good society. When rights are assumed to be basic there seems to be no way to avoid an arbitrariness in the list of alleged rights and/or how conflicts of rights can be adjudicated. For claims to rights to be intelligible, they must be correlative to specific contexts and institutions we believe serve a common good. If families, for example, have rights, they do so because such rights are the means to protect the goods we believe constitutive of the family.

But when rights are taken to be the fundamental moral reality we are encouraged to take an ultimately degrading perspective on society. No real society can *exist* when its citizens' only way of relating is in terms of noninterference. The language of "rights," especially as it is displayed by liberal political theory, encourages us to live as if we had no common interests or beliefs. We are thus trained to regard even our children as potential strangers from whom we need protection. But this is a formula for the disintegration of society as well as the disintegration of the moral self, as it trains us to pursue our interests as ends in themselves.

Therefore, even though I do not reject all use of rights language, as a basic moral language, I find it insufficient on grounds of social theory. Secondly, however, it may not be a case of whether rights language in and of itself is appropriate but whether such language is overused or used in inappropriate contexts. I have tried to suggest that there are good reasons for thinking that it is an overused language in our society and that, in particular, it does not apply to the familial context.

Thirdly, there is the question of whether rights language, even if appropriate, can be applied to children. For "rights" presupposes a moral psychology which, some have argued, at least very young children fail to meet. I have no wish to enter into this argument here, as I think it would serve little purpose. However, it should be pointed out that if rights are to be claimed for very young children, counter-arguments must be provided against those who argue that young children have neither the rational capacity nor the "interests" necessary to have rights.

I must mention that I regard this last issue as a category mistake. Morally the question is not what claim children have on us, but what our responsibility is to them, irrespective of their ability to make a "claim."

I expect that the language of rights will still hold great attraction for members of this commission. It is the historic language of our society and any policy decision seems more persuasive when framed in its terms. Also, as I have suggested, rights language in today's social context appears to serve the child's interest. Moreover, if I have been at least partly right, my argument would seem to require the commission to appeal to a normative conception of the family which not all in our society could support. Quite properly then, many on the commission must wonder if they have the moral grounds to take that kind of position. The language of rights appears as a compromise that diverse groups can interpret in their own way. However, if the commission decides to use the language of rights, I hope that such language is employed with qualification.

Autonomy, Paternalism, and the Care of Children

Because we tend to approach issues such as experimentation armed only with the language of rights, we cannot help but distort the complexity of the issue. The only question at stake is whether the proposed research violates the autonomy of the subject of the research. In particular, both in terms of therapy and experimentation, it is argued we must avoid taking a paternalistic attitude toward the research subject. Paternalism (or maternalism) is always viewed negatively on the assumption that our relation to one another should be one of complete independence. Such an ideal is supported by the psychological fact that those who try to "help" the sick or the young often do so as a means of gaining and holding power. Thus "rights" are attributed to children in the hopes of securing for them some of the power their parents possess.

But surely this is a formula for the destruction of the child—that is, it is to turn the child into an adult. The child's need for trust, love, and care cannot be filled by giving the child rights. I am aware that those recommending "rights" language as a means to protect children from parents who neither love their children nor can be trusted not to harm them do so exactly because there seems to be no other alternative. But we cannot protect children by denying that children rightly need to be treated maternally.

Indeed it is my contention there is nothing wrong with paternalism or maternalism once we see that the development of autonomous beings is not the culmination of the moral life. Rather the goal of parenting is the creation of people who can enter into trustful relations because they have learned not to fear the other as a threat to their "autonomy." To be sure, such people have the capacity of self-determination, but this capacity is not the same as being "autonomous." It is rather the ability to receive as well as to give without using receiving or giving as a means to control the other.

To make these remarks more concrete, let me again call your attention to the more traditional form of family. We tend to think that the idea of raising children to be autonomous is an objective value to which all rational people should adhere. But think of Orthodox Jews. They are not raising their children to be autonomous, if that means that when they reach the age of reason they can choose whether or not to become a Jew. To think of being or not being a Jew as a matter of choice is already to betray the tradition. Rather they raise their children to become the best that they know—namely, Jews.

To call such a process "paternalism" in a negative sense is simply question begging and special pleading. It is not a question of paternalism but parental responsibility to initiate their children into the best form of life that they know. Not to do so would be either cowardice or irresponsibility. Caring for children both in terms of their health and their education is not a question of paternalism, but of what kind of responsibilities parents should have, given the expectations of the community in which both the parents and child exist.

In this respect the claim that parents often do not know what is best for their children and that children are capable of making sensible decisions for themselves is simply beside the point. It is of course true that some parents, irrespective of what community they are part of, do not know what is best for their children. The important claim is that they *should know* what is best for their children in matters of importance. No doubt many Orthodox Jewish children do not feel it is in their best interest to be Orthodox Jews, but that is not relevant to the issue. On important matters children simply do not have interests until they have been taught what interests to have.

Nor should this position be interpreted as denying all respect and moral standing for children. It is simply not the case that our respect for a child's status is dependent on whether the child does or does not have "rights." A "right" is not the same as a "standing" that requires respect. Indeed in traditional Jewish families the child is highly respected and honored exactly by being treated as a participant in the community—that is, as being able to perform his or her function as a fellow Jew.

Thus, in spite of its prevalence today, the issue of paternalism is a misleading way to state the moral issue of parental responsibility to care for and nurture children. To be a parent is to perform an office for a community of seeing that the child finds his or her way to the moral best that the community has to offer. Of course, the parent does not, or should not, have complete power over the child, since the child also has a standing in the community apart from the parent. Such a standing cannot be guaranteed by the language of rights but depends on the moral substance of that community and how it has learned to regard children as valuable beings.

Respect for Persons, Covenants, and Proxy Consent

The different kind of perspective I have developed for issues raised by experimentation on children can be illustrated by commenting on Dr. William Bartholome's position [1]. Though I am critical of the way Dr. Bartholome argues, I am sympathetic to many of his conclusions. I will try to show, therefore, that his conclusions do not require, and in fact may even be undercut by, his use of the language of rights and respect for person *qua* person.

Dr. Bartholome begins by defining a child as a person below the age of fourteen to sixteen. As I suggested above, this kind of designation of children assumes that whether someone is or is not a child is an empirical question. But this is clearly mistaken. "Child" is a notion that first requires conceptual and moral analysis in order even to know what empirical characteristics will count as locating a child. The "age of reason" criteria suffers from the same confusion. This is not to argue for a functional understanding of children (a child is only such in relation to certain assumed tasks or relations), but it is to suggest that often our presuppositions regarding what a child is rest on unexamined premises. If we do not raise this kind of question, we are apt to forget that morally "childhood" is dependent on our understanding of family and community.

Dr. Bartholome argues that consent is the primary moral issue in determining the morality or immorality of experimentation on children. However this position is somewhat qualified, as he claims that consent is never a sufficient condition to justify medical intervention or experimentation. But he seems to assume that, while not a *sufficient* condition, consent remains a *necessary* condition for any therapy or research. He does so by appealing to Paul Ramsey's attempt to base consent in the "canon of loyalty" between physician and patient. Yet Ramsey's own position in this respect is less than clear. Ramsey appeals to the Jewish and Christian sense of "covenant" to provide a paradigm of his "canon of loyalty," but it is not clear how the analogy between God's covenant with his people and the "canon of loyalty" between doctor and patient is justified or illuminating.

Like Ramsey, Dr. Bartholome also appeals to consent as a necessary correlative of our respect for "persons." But the Kantian sense of "respect for persons" seems to be committed to a more individualistic conception of human dignity than the communitarian conception of "covenant" can allow. To be a member of a covenant is to be loyal to the commitments of a community in a manner that renders suspect the placing of individual interests before those of the community and the object of loyalty that the community serves. In other words, I am suggesting that Dr. Bartholome may have some difficulty having his covenant and Kant too.

Dr. Bartholome also suggests that the opaqueness of others and the humility appropriate toward others' interests are reasons making consent imperative for any medical intervention. However this is a pragmatic justification and suggests that if the opaqueness is removed, as it might be in certain cases, then consent can be overridden by other interests. I raise this issue because I think Dr. Bartholome's paper illustrates the general ambiguity concerning why consent is made the central issue for medical intervention. I do not wish to argue that consent is unimportant; I am simply suggesting that, in spite of the fact that it is assumed to be central, no convincing arguments have been established. Without a clear sense of what kind of justification should be given for consent, we cannot anticipate how consent should be institutionalized within medical practice and research.

It is my hunch that consent has become central for us, not because it is a fundamental category, but because in a liberal society it is the only way we have to protect ourselves from one another. In other words, without denying that consent in any society has some moral force, I suspect that its moral force in our society arises as much from political reasons as from moral ones.

Until this is clarified I think the issue of proxy consent must remain confused. I would at least suggest that proxy consent, which Dr. Bartholome interprets to be primarily an attempt to protect the child, can equally be seen as an attempt to protect the integrity of the family unit. In other words, proxy consent as an institution is one way to insure that whatever is done to the child is done in accordance with the moral convictions and traditions of that family. The problem is that proxy consent in our society has become a power in the hands of certain parents whom we fear have corrupt moral convictions about the kind of care that should or should not be given to children.

This is, of course, the basis of Dr. Bartholome's criticism of those defenses of proxy consent in the nontherapeutic context. Though Bartholome does not develop it, I suspect that he could make much more of the difficulty of distinguishing between therapeutic and nontherapeutic contexts. He suggests that this is an extremely difficult distinction to draw in practice. His judgment can be amply documented — for example, in the treatment of young children suffering from leukemia; it is by no means clear when treatment for one child conforms or does not conform to "established and accepted medical practices." This problem is occasioned not simply by the doctor's need to learn more to help future patients, but by the fact that every patient is different in a way that makes "standard" practices suspect for that patient. (For an extraordinary depiction of the bind parents are caught in when they subject their children to extraordinary therapies in the hope it may do "some good," see Peter DeVries' novel *The Blood of the Lamb*.)

Generally, I think that Dr. Bartholome's criticisms of proxy consent in nontherapeutic contexts are correct, but Bartholome's own position betrays some of the same tendencies of those who defend proxy consent — for instance, to say that children can participate in "nonrisk" experiments because it will contribute to their moral growth. Does Dr. Bartholome believe we can ask children to participate in nontherapeutic experiments even if such participation would be morally supererogatory?

Those who argue that we can choose to involve children in such research do so by appealing to the common good. But such appeals are too vague because they seem to imply that there are some things we can expect children to do for the good of the greatest number. Such arguments then would appear very similar to utilitarian arguments that seem contradicted by the very moral presuppositions that sustain our commitment to informed consent.

In response those who defend proxy consent can take an entirely different tact. We can consent for the child on the assumption, in certain contexts, that we know what the child ought to choose for himself or herself — e.g., self-preservation and health — irrespective of the interests of the community. I think that Bartholome's worry that we cannot know the child's real interest is beside the point. Defenders of proxy consent are not claiming that we know this individual child's interest, but rather than we know generally certain basic goods that all people have in common (not the same as "the common good") which we can act on with assurance.

However this argument still proves less than convincing because of the vagueness of terms such as *self-preservation* and *health*. Morally we do not choose to survive as an end in itself but because survival provides the conditions for the achievement of other moral ends. The question is whether children are not, like adults, forced at times "to choose" between those ends that we survive for and survival. I suspect good communities assume that children are those who should be protected from having to make that choice as long as possible. (This may be why we want to use rights language — that is, to remind ourselves that children require special protection. Unfortunately, however, the language of rights has become an end in itself rather than a reminder of why we wish to protect children in the first place.) However that does mean that at times it may be necessary to make the decision for the child—e.g., in the case of the Orthodox Jew, that it is better to die as a Jew than to be raised as a Gentile.

This indicates that children, even infants, can have a moral role in a community even before they are agents. Dr. Bartholome would make a child's contribution to a community dependent on his or her maturation level (surely an important criterion), but I am suggesting that sometimes communities can choose in a morally humane manner to assume that the child has moral standing in the community even when the child cannot choose that standing on his own. Formally this position bears some similarity to those who defend proxy consent in terms of the common good, but in contrast to such appeals I think that there is no way to determine what interests the child should have as a member of the human community *qua* human community. As humans we share a moral capacity and needs, but such capacity and needs are not sufficient to ground concrete moral judgments; that requires the convictions and practices of specific actual communities.

My argument can be illustrated by noting Bartholome's criticism of the assertion that we all have a responsibility to participate in nontherapeutic research. Bartholome suggests that this judgment proceeds from the unwarranted assumption that we have a moral obligation to perform acts of supererogation. However there is no *a priori* way to draw a distinction between practices that are obligatory and those that are supererogatory. Such distinctions depend on the concrete convictions and practices of particular communities. If medical research plays a crucial role in advancing the primary purposes of a community, then the assumption that everyone should participate in that research may make sense. I suspect, however, that it cannot be sustained in our society. As a result Dr. Bartholome's conclusion certainly seems warranted, especially since we have no reason to subject some to undue risks now in order that future generations will be free of certain kinds of diseases.

If the position I have been trying to develop is at least partially correct, however, Dr. Bartholome's appeal to the Kantian notion that we should always treat another as an end and never as a means is too simply stated. The question is never whether we use another as a means, but whether the end is commensurate with the person's good as a member of a morally healthy community. Nor is it sufficient to say that we ought to treat others as persons—that is, as ends in themselves. For example, Dr. Bartholome suggests not to require the parents to repair their infant's club feet would be violating the "infant as a person." But the issue is not really whether the infant is being treated as a person but whether, given what we know about how important it is to walk, we think that such parents are providing proper care. In other words such a decision is dependent on our normative understanding of the kind of care parents ought to give children in order to secure as satisfying a life for them as is possible.

Appeals to the notion of "person" as a way to underscore parents' obligations to their children is therefore unnecessary, if not misleading. It simply introduces the question of whether children are persons — and that is a misleading question. We care for children because they are children, not because they are persons.

A similar kind of problem is involved in Dr. Bartholome's appeal to rights language. I don't necessarily disagree with his position, but I simply do not think he needs rights language to make it work. In fact, it is difficult to know exactly what he means by "rights." He sometimes speaks as if rights are correlative to our "membership in the human community," but then he suggests that rights require a community with "certain constitutive characteristics." It may be that Dr. Bartholome can have it both ways on this matter, but if so he must be able to spell out how a particular community's characteristics are dependent on our membership in the "human community."

Or again he argues that rights language makes sense as a way to indicate that an infant has a claim to be fed, have adequate shelter, and have other basic needs met. In other words, the infant has claims over against his or her parents to provide for the infant's needs. If the parents cannot do so, then the state can step in to see that the infant is cared for, either by aiding the parents or by seeing that the infant is cared for by others who will meet those needs. I have no objection in principle to rights language being used in this manner if it is clearly seen as dependent on the more basic language of parental obligation. In other words such "rights" are simply ways to mark off basic parental roles and obligations that the state can expect any parent, regardless of their peculiar convictions or practices, to meet.

However Dr. Bartholome obviously has a more substantive claim in mind, for he argues that these role-dependent rights are dependent on what H. L. A. Hart calls "general rights." In Dr. Bartholome's words, "the infant must be recognized to have the right to be treated as a member of the human community, as a person." But as I have tried to suggest, being morally a member of the human community, even with a dime, will not buy you a cup of coffee. The recognition and respect due infants and children are not insured by posing their "rights" as members of the human community, but by their existence in the kind of community that has learned to value children as members of that community.

On the same grounds Dr. Bartholome also argues that an infant has a right to the care a physician can give. I find this an extremely doubtful assertion, as the mere existence of doctors does not mean that each individual infant has a claim on their care (which of course raises the further question as to the extent of care that can be claimed). It seems best to see the care that the physician is obligated to give as an extension of the parent's basic responsibilities. In other words, contrary to Bartholome's suggestion, the infant does not have a direct claim on the doctor, but rather has a claim on the doctor as mediated through the responsibilities of the parents.

Dr. Bartholome is concerned that infants and children have a basis for being treated with respect and care. But I think that Dr. Bartholome fails to specify what normative conception of family and community makes such respect morally compelling. His position requires that children be turned into potential adults in order to be respected, but that is to fail to treat them for what they are—namely, children.

For example, Dr. Bartholome suggests that since the "end of parenting is formation of highly developed persons, i.e., persons who are free, autonomous beings capable of reasoned choices, it is essential that infants and children be treated as persons." But again it seems to me that this posits a morally false sense of autonomy on which our respect and treatment of children depends. This poses some difficult problems in respect to children who are retarded, because they will never be able to achieve the kind of autonomy that Dr. Bartholome thinks crucial to being and becoming a "person."

Dr. Bartholome thinks that unless the "rights of infants and children" can be established on the grounds of their membership in the human species, then there is no way to justify intervention on behalf of abused or neglected children. But as I suggested above, such intervention does not require a doctrine of the rights of the child against the parents, but a normative conception of parenting and the family.

That does not mean parents own their children; rather they have responsibilities that are correlative to their community's sense of the importance of children.

Conclusion

In spite of my criticism of Dr. Bartholome, I think he is grappling with issues that are well nigh insoluble in our cultural situation. No philosophical device, whether it be in the language of rights or some other alternative, is sufficient to lead us out of this dilemma. We live at a time when we are simply not clear about why we should have children or what we should do with them once we have them, and talk of formal "rights" will not provide the answer.

In traditional religious communities it was claimed that children were a gift of God. They were neither the property of their parents nor of the community. Rather parents and community were but the way God's care was mediated to the child.

With the loss of that sense of providence the child became the possession of the parent for, after all, it was by the sheer exertion of parental will that the child had existence at all. Such "paternalism" could be extremely beneficial to children, but at the same time it always contained the potential for despotism and arbitrariness.

A natural way to place a check on the unbalanced power of the parent was to assume that if God does not own the child, and the parents do not own the child, then the child must own himself (or, alternatively, that the state must own the child). But what all of this ignores is that it is not a question of ownership at all, but rather whether we should be the kind of people who can welcome new life among us even when such life is destined to change our own. The language of rights, I suspect, will teach us little about the kind of skills we need to train ourselves to take on that kind of task.

I have been able to write with more freedom than the commission can have in formulating its policy. I can write as if an ideal world is possible, but you cannot. I can write as if experimentation on and with children might be a possibility if certain assumptions about parenting and community are present, but you cannot. Moreover I have suggested that the most readily available language in our society to deal with these matters has some definite drawbacks. I frankly do not know what kind of policy I would recommend if I were on the commission.

However I think I would at least try to write the report in a manner that manifests the moral uncertainty with which we are faced. Too often our ethics and our policies are formed as if we are clearer than in fact we are. By stating the issue ambiguously, at least you could signal to the research community, the government, and the parents that make up the American people that morally we are not O.K. when it comes to our assumptions about the place and role of children in our society. In such a situation it does not seem to be an unwarranted conclusion that if we are to experiment on children, it must be very, very carefully. A more radical suggestion would be, that in the light of our moral unclarity, which after all is not just a problem of theory but of ourselves, we should not use children in nontherapeutic experimentation. Or finally, it might be interesting to say only the broadest guidelines can be drawn and that the justification of each experiment depends greatly on how the experimenters can morally articulate their purpose as a way to serve particular people (the health of the nation will not do) and why the children and parents of the experiment have a stake in that purpose. It is just as important that protocols be moral documents, not only in the sense of consent, as that they show that the experiment is scientifically well conceived. Protocols, like judicial decisions, should have moral dicta which show us how they are justified in the light of our basic convictions.

NOTE

1. This was a paper prepared for the National Commission for the Protection of Human Subjects of Biomedical and Behavioral Research. I was asked in particular to respond to papers by Drs. Donald Worsfold and William Bartholome, who had prepared earlier papers for the commission. Dr. Worsfold's paper was never published, but Dr. Bartholome's paper along with my response can be found in William Bartholome, "The Ethics on Nontherapeutic Clinical Research on Children," and "Proxy Consent in the Medical Context: The Infant as Person," in *Research Involving Children*, Washington, D.C.: DHEW Publication No. (OS) 77-0005, essay no. 3. Because Dr. Worsfold's paper has not been published I have edited or omitted most of my comments about his position.

8

Theological Reflection
on *In Vitro* Fertilization

Theology, Ethics, and *In Vitro* Fertilization

I am honored to be asked to testify before the Ethics Advisory Board of the Department of Health, Education, and Welfare about the ethical questions raised by *in vitro* fertilization. Even more, I appreciate that I have been invited to speak from a theological perspective, for that is what I care most about. Though I have been trained as an "ethicist" and my work is usually classified as "ethics," I understand myself to be a theologian.[1] Yet I must warn you that to seriously address the issue of *in vitro* fertilization from a theological perspective will require me to raise issues that may seem irrelevant to your task of developing principles determining the public policy of the nation.

For by speaking from a theological perspective I do not pretend to speak from principles that are or should be shared by everyone in our society. You should also know that my own methodological presuppositions in this respect are not widely shared among those who work in theological ethics. Rather it is most often assumed that theological ethics must develop arguments that should compel consent from all rational subjects, irrespective of their religious convictions or lack of religious convictions. Of course, that results in the somewhat ironical state of affairs that committees such as this invite representatives of religious communities to show how their communities' particular convictions throw light on an issue, only to be told that a Christian's views on the subject are not necessarily related to their religious convictions. Christian ethicists therefore say what any right-thinking person or moral philosopher would say.

Well, I simply do not believe such should be the case. It will be the heart of my argument that theological beliefs *do* make a difference

142

for how *in vitro* fertilization is understood. But since my own views are correlative to my theological convictions it raises the issue of how seriously the committee can take them for consideration of public policy.

It is my own view that the presumed moral agreement or consensus among many philosophical and religious ethicists is unfounded. Such agreement can be maintained only by providing an account of morality so formal that it cannot possibly have any normative implications. In fact I take the moral challenge of our time to be the recognition that we live amid "fragments" of past moral positions, none of which can claim our loyalty on grounds of rationality in itself.[2] In such a situation, by taking seriously the particularity of Christian convictions perhaps I can at least help clarify the difficulty of formulating public policy where it involves moral issues.

After having made this strong claim about the dependence of my argument on theological presuppositions, however, I must tell you that there is no *direct* connection between theological beliefs and the question of the permissibility or impermissibility of *in vitro* fertilization. There is nothing in Scripture that says "You shall not commit *in vitro* fertilization"; nor do I think you can show any direct connection between theological assertions about God's creative and redemptive purposes and *in vitro* fertilization. There may be theologians who think this can be done, but I am skeptical whether they can make such arguments work.

Rather, to understand the relationship between theological claims and questions about *in vitro* fertilization, I must ask you to suspend some of the usual notions about religious belief and how it relates to the moral life. The primary function of religious belief is not to describe the world or to determine the rightness or wrongness of particular actions, but to form a community that understands itself as having a particular mission in the world. To be sure, that mission involves beliefs about the nature of the world and what one should and should not do, but those judgments are mediated by the practices that have been established as essential to being a people of a particular sort. Put starkly, for the Christian the question of the use or non-use of *in vitro* fertilization will be determined primarily by whether such a procedure is appropriate to our understanding of what kind of community we should be and in particular what kind of attitudes about parenting we should foster. In other words, it is not a question of whether *in vitro* fertilization is right or wrong, but a practical judgment of whether this kind of technique furthers or is compatible with our community's understanding of itself. Issues such as *in vitro* fertilization are fundamentally symbolic in that they are primarily determined by the wisdom of a community.

Ethically, this means that religious convictions are not usually of the sort that determine whether something is right or wrong in itself, but rather they determine what *we* should be. I have argued elsewhere that contemporary ethics has been too concerned with "quandaries" or decisions and has failed to pay sufficient attention to the notion that what we *are* is as important as what we do.[3] From such a perspective questions concerning the morality of *in vitro* fertilization cannot be determined in isolation from the implications of its use for the character of the Christian community and individuals.

Christian Parenting and *In Vitro* Fertilization

In his testimony before the committee, Leon Kass has rightly argued the first question to ask is not whether *in vitro fertilization* is right or wrong, but what is it? [4]. He argues that we should first try to understand what we are doing when we seek to develop *in vitro* fertilization techniques. My emphasis is a bit different from his, however, as he wants to understand the procedure of *in vitro* fertilization and I want to begin still another step back and look at why we feel the need to develop such a procedure. Is it simply the result of humankind's continuing quest to understand ourselves better through science? Or does it derive from our pledge to care for one another through the office of medicine by alleviating unnecessary physical hindrances to our moral projects? Or is this procedure a mark of our sinful pretension to insure immortality through biological continuity?

My first question then is not one of decision but how to understand such a procedure in a manner that gives direction to a community's moral project. When put in this context I assume that possible misuse of the procedure is not the primary question, as every invention of man is open to perversion. The question is whether there can be a moral determination of when it should not be used.

To make this way of proceeding more concrete, I want to direct your attention to a childless couple who have come to their minister for counseling about their wish to have children. (I will have to assume that this is a minister who failed to take his course in psychological counseling in seminary and therefore still thinks that Christian convictions should have something to do with how he talks with and even, in a moment of bravery, advises this couple.) How should the minister or the couple, as Christians, understand the importance of having children and, in particular, their own biological children?

In other words, the question to begin with is why anyone should want to have children in the first place. We assume that such a desire is not arbitrary but based on our most profound moral convictions. Yet it has been my experience that when you ask people why they want children they usually become surprisingly inarticulate. They say it is fun (obviously these have never had children), that it is a manifestation of their love (but then what do you do with your children if the love fades), or it is to please the grandparents or to prevent the couple from being lonely (again less than good reasons, since then the child is being used for some purpose other than him- or herself), or that children are our hope for the future (and then they always disappoint us).

I am well aware that part of the hesitancy stems from the fact that the question seems illegitimate. And indeed I suppose it is; most of the time we simply do not have to think very much about such matters. The very institutions of culture carry obvious expectations which make such questions seem irrelevant. But perhaps procedures such as *in vitro* fertilization are so troubling for us because they are occurring exactly at a time when our institutions do not seem to have much assuredness. In doubt as to why we are having children or what we ought to do with them once we have had them, we feel more secure not raising these questions, on the assumption that the unexamined life is indeed worth living. But these unexamined questions are at the heart of the issues raised by *in vitro* fertilization.

Presupposed in the therapeutic justification of *in vitro* fertilization is the assumption that biology has some extremely important role to play in parenting. That does seem obvious, since biological pregnancy is the necessary condition for parenting. Beyond that obvious fact, does the demand of couples to have their own biological children suggest that in the absence of any deeper understanding of parenting our last resort is biology? No one would wish to deny the importance of the experience of pregnancy, but is it so important that we should be willing to expend huge amounts of time and money to provide it?

Also involved in the development of this technique is a peculiar sort of biological determinism. Often those who defend the technique in order to give women the experience of pregnancy see nothing wrong with the further use of the technique through surrogate mothers. At once the technique is defended in the name of the crucial relation between biology and parenting, and then a form of parenting is defended that seems to make biological parenting secondary.

Indeed, the way critics of *in vitro* fertilization raise the spector of surrogate motherhood strikes me as but another indication that we are less than clear about what moral role parenting involves. The critics seem to assume that obviously most people would agree that surrogate motherhood is a bad idea. Why should people think that? They condemn the idea of one woman paying another to carry her genetic child and thus avoiding the trouble and danger of pregnancy. But surrogate motherhood should not be condemned because it is open to commercial distortion or because it might involve attitudes on the part of the "nonpregnant" mother which we usually feel are incompatible with the willingness to have and raise children. Surely it is possible to conceive of a woman carrying another woman's child out of friendship when the latter is incapable of carrying her child. Confronted with that kind of case, I suspect our problem is not that we know what is wrong with surrogate motherhood, but we have no idea *why* we should think it right or wrong, and thus we become dogmatic about its "wrongness".

I mention these issues not to argue that *in vitro* fertilization is wrong, but only to suggest that morally it calls forward our most profound assumptions about the role of parenting and how that role is formed by the good ends of particular communities. Because our culture is currently at a loss to give direction to the institution of parenting, *in vitro* fertilization is troubling and we cannot articulate why we have developed it. For example, I suspect that the response of most people when they first think about *in vitro* fertilization is not an "ethical" judgment at all; it is simply that such a technique seems bizarre. We tend to think of the bizarre as an esthetic category having no ethical significance, but I think that is a mistake. For what is bizarre about *in vitro* fertilization is how a civilization that has approved of people aborting all unwanted children can at the same time sponsor an extraordinary technique to allow a few women to have the experience of pregnancy. Or that a civilization that has been told that we are overpopulated and on the brink of ecological disaster has developed such a technique. What this indicates to me is not that we have a corrupt civilization but that we have one that has no way of providing an understanding of what any of us are doing when we have (or don't have) children.

But we must come back to our minister counseling the childless couple. All I have tried to establish at this point is whatever the minister says to the couple necessarily will involve assumptions about why they are having children in the first place. Though it is true that Christians and non-Christians alike have children, it is not clear that morally they are doing the same thing. As I have tried to suggest, having children is not a natural fact or a necessity, but draws on our deepest assumptions about the nature of our existence.[4]

Therefore, for Christians, having children must be placed in the context of some very substantive claims about the nature of the world and God's relation to it. You will have to forgive me if some of what follows sounds homiletic, but there is no other way to say it. Christians believe that the world is deeply bent by sin, most poignantly manifest in the distrust that characterizes all relations between people. Violence and coercion are not accidental to such a world but are integral to its nature. For example, from our perspective people are not racist because they are ignorant, but racism is a manifestation of fear, fueled by the corrupt and prideful assumption that the only way to get out of this life alive is by taking control of our existence. In other words, we believe that distrust and untruthfulness present among us are but the inevitable consequences of a world built on the assumption that men, not God, rule.

The Christian and the Jew believe that they have been given a special mission in such a world. Namely, they have been called to form communities that manifest the trust and love possible between people when they recognize the sovereignty of God over all life. To be sure, they are often unfaithful to the task, but even their unfaithfulness points to the kind of life that should be possible between people.

In the context of this view, the business of having children has particular moral significance, for children are the sign that hope is stronger than despair—and remember, Christians believe that there is plenty to despair about in the world. Please note: I am not suggesting that Christians believe that our hope is in our children, as that would be blasphemy, but that our children are a sign of the kind of hope our faith in God gives us.

Put differently, children serve to anchor us to history. The temptation for Christians is to always think that God's salvation is beyond time or at least abstracted from time. Through our obligation to have children Christians are bound in time as they form communities that make clear their conviction that God is working in the world to form a kingdom of peace and justice. Thus our commitment, indeed obligation, to have children is our pledge that our salvation is not ahistorical but takes place through the contingencies of history.

Now you may well think you do not need all this theological exposition to make a very simple point. After all, to quote Auden, "Existentialists declare / That they are in complete despair, / Yet go on having children" (*Under Which Lyre*). I certainly do not intend to imply that the views about children I have explicated here are limited only to Christians; rather I am simply trying to say what I take Christian conviction to entail.

However, there is another aspect of the Christian view that is not so obvious. The central documents of the Christian faith, which, oddly enough, have very little to say about sex, family, or children, do not make marriage and the family the first form of life. The Christians from whom we get the New Testament seem to have thought that the demands of the kingdom were such that the single life was at least equally valid. Therefore, it was not incumbent on every Christian to marry or have children, since, after all, the community was primarily to grow through conversion of those outside it. Put simply, Christians broke the assumption that marriage was a natural or moral necessity and thus made it a vocation. (And a vocation is not something you choose, but that to which you are called.) They had to think about why they were having children, because their own beliefs now convinced them they were not obliged. I realize this will come as a great shock to those Christians today who assume that the truthfulness of Christianity depends on how well it reinforces their natural and cultural assumptions, but that is no great matter. As Chesterton pointed out, Christianity has not failed, it has just seldom been tried.

Christians assume that having children is not simply a natural event, but one dependent on their deepest convictions. For example, many fail to notice that past condemnation of contraception, which some take to be an unwarranted imposition of biological necessity, was in its cultural context the attempt to take procreation out of the natural realm and subject it to the realm of freedom. For from such a perspective children are not chosen, but viewed as the natural benefits that result from the obligations of those called to marriage. Children are thus viewed as gifts necessary to sustain a people whose task is to witness to the sovereignty of a God in a world that knows him not. We, therefore, are called upon to have children, even though we know we cannot guarantee their safety.

All of this may still seem miles away from the question of *in vitro* fertilization, but I think it is relevant. As the minister counsels the childless couple, it is reasonable for him to try to help them find ways to have children. But the question is, how hard should they try? Nothing in the Christian attitude toward parenting requires that parenting should be defined biologically. Surely, before you ask medicine and science to develop techniques to allow you to have *your* biological children, it should be determined why it is so important that they be "biologically" yours. And as I suggested above, the couple must realize that Christians do not assume that having children is a necessity for everyone in their community.

Moreover, it is not as if a childless couple among Christians is bereft of all forms and experiences of parenting. If being a parent is first of all an office of a community, rather than a description of a biological process, even those without immediate children still have "parental responsibilities." Every community depends on educators, doctors, and countless other roles directly related to and in support of the community's commitment to its children. I am not trying to suggest that such activity is the same as responsibility for a particular child, but neither is it irrelevant for how one might understand one's parental responsibilities.

Even more important for Christians, given the specific commands for them to be concerned with widows and orphans and their responsibility to welcome the stranger among them, adoption surely seems to be the most appropriate strategy for childlessness. I seriously doubt, therefore, that Christian convictions about parenting can supply the kind of intelligibility necessary to make the development of *in vitro* fertilization morally explicable. In particular, Christians must surely be doubtful of any moral defenses of *in vitro* fertilization that claim this technique as an extension of freedom from natural necessity. From our perspective such a claim involves the pretentious assumption that there is no limit to the right of people to perpetuate themselves.

Biology and Parenthood

The position I have developed may sound particularly strange coming from a Christian, for many of the Christian critiques of *in vitro* fertilization have seemed to assume that the technique was wrong because it was "unnatural." Thus Ramsey has argued

> we procreate new beings like ourselves in the midst of our love for one another, and in this there is a trace of the original mystery by which God created the world because of His love. God created nothing apart from His love; and without the divine love was not anything made that was made. Neither should there be among men and women . . . any love set out of the context of responsibility for procreation, any begetting apart from the sphere of love. A reflection of God's love, binding himself to the world and the world to himself, is found in the claim He placed upon men and women in their creation when He bound the nurturing of marital love and procreation together in the nature of human sexuality. Thus, the Christian understanding of life stems from the second article of the Creed, not from the first or from facts of nature; and this is the source of the Christian knowledge that men and women should not put radically asunder what God joined together in creation. Thus a Christian, as such, intends the world as God intends the world . . . . And in human procreativity out of the depths of human sexual love is prefigured God's own act of creation out of the profound mystery of his love revealed in Christ. To put radically asunder what God joined together in parenthood when He made love procreative, to procreate from beyond the sphere of love (AID, for example, or making human life in a test-tube), or to posit acts of sexual love beyond the sphere of responsible procreation (by definition, marriage), means a refusal of the image of God's creation in our own. ([7], pp. 38-39)

Ramsey's view seems committed to the view that sexual intercourse is the only way Christians should try to become parents. But such a conclusion seems too strong even on Ramsey's grounds. For as Ramsey notes biology is never simply biology, but the appeal to the "natural" way is but a form of human intentionality. In other words, one can never just have sex as if it is a natural given, but rather all sex is "unnatural" insofar as it is formed by human intentions. Yet even on a strict reading of "biological reproduction," it remains unclear why

Ramsey would exclude *in vitro* fertilization on these grounds, since it can, as Toulmin [8] has recently suggested, be interpreted as an extension of what we are already doing through artificial insemination by the husband (both being attempts to aid couples to produce *their* biological children.)

I suspect that Ramsey has already anticipated the force of that objection and that is why he has not made such appeals in his testimony before this committee [6]. Instead, he emphasizes the possibility of damage to the fetus and child and the assault such a procedure represents against the family, and women in particular. Ramsey's arguments in this respect are an attempt to find grounds for saying *in vitro* fertilization represents or involves inherently wrong behavior. Underlying his arguments, however, I suspect is profound doubt whether our culture, in the absence of any shared assumptions about the place of children in our lives, has the wisdom to control such a technique. In other words, Ramsey's search for a knockdown argument against *in vitro* fertilization in terms of harm to the conception is an attempt to take the issue out of the realm of judgment, as he fears we lack the wisdom as a society to utilize this technology in a morally worthy manner. In this respect, I think Ramsey may well be right that the very development of such a technique indicates that as a culture we lack an appropriate sense of parenting to guide its use, apart from any moral determination regarding the laboratory technique in itself.

I suspect also that Ramsey's strategy is a conscious attempt to find arguments that will serve as secular analogues for his religious conviction about parenting. His religious assumption — "what God has joined together let no man put asunder" — cannot and ought not be made the basis of public policy. As a result he resorts to liberal arguments concerning harm and "informed consent," since it seems clear that *in vitro* fertilization violates both. For all of Ramsey's polemical brilliance, I think it fairly obvious that he has not shown that the "harm" or potential "harm" involved in *in vitro* fertilization renders the procedure inherently immoral; nor has he shown how the condition of "informed consent" has been violated.

Having thus criticized Ramsey, I must admit that I think there is much wisdom in his understanding of the importance of the "biological" context of parenthood. For sex within the proper context may in fact be an important condition for the development of the intimate bond we think significant to prepare us to claim our children as our own. His mistake is to argue that it is the *necessary* condition for such claiming. We forget that one of the great moral advances of our civilization is in parents' willingness to claim their children as their own. One of the most difficult tasks of any culture is encouraging males to accept responsibility for their children. Ramsey may well be right that once procreation is severed from sexual intercourse the basis for accepting the responsibility for parenthood becomes problematic. At the very least, once that separation has occurred, some very substantive convictions are needed to direct us to have appropriate attitudes toward those beings who present themselves to us as our children.

Indeed, as I have tried to suggest above, it is exactly because Christians broke with the prevailing idea of procreation as a natural and moral necessity, that their own commitments to children become so important. They learned children were not *theirs* but God's. Therefore, not even biology could determine ownership, as children were not theirs to own. Rather they find themselves pledged to their children because of the depth of their conviction about the God who has called them into being. But if our culture no longer views the having of children in such terms, Ramsey is no doubt right to think that *in vitro* fertilization is particularly problematic in such a situation.

I do not wish to deny the importance of biology in providing the medium for "bonding" between mother and child. I cannot, however, accept the crude determinism that assumes that when "bonding" has not occurred through nine months of pregnancy, mother and child are both under a decisive disadvantage. Biology may help us learn to be parents, but we also must be guided by a moral portrayal of parenting that cannot be biologically derived.

There is a new movement in the public schools to educate our youth about "parenting." The secular criteria for good parenting cannot possibly take account of the foregoing description of responsibility to God in the roles we assume as parents, yet the biological description is insufficient. It will be extremely interesting to see what moral presuppositions will inform programs aimed at "educating future parents." I suspect the general approach will be "if you want to have children, then this is the way to be fairly successful at it," thus assuming that the reason to have children is a "private" matter not open to moral discourse. Rather all that matters is that one be emotionally and materially prepared for the "responsibility."[5]

Medicine, Science, and Religion

One reasonable response to the kind of position I develop is to say: "All this is simply beside the point. What we are talking about is not philosophical or theological presumptions behind parenting. We are talking about the development of a technique derived from medicine's traditional commitment to alleviate the distress of patients. Some women cannot have children because of blocked fallopian tubes. All we are trying to do is provide them with the means to reproduce. Surely you Christians, in spite of your odd views about parenting, see the value in a doctor trying to help people do what an accident of nature prevents them from doing."

In brief, my first reaction to this response is to ask if the assumptions about the aim of medicine are in fact correct. Is the task of medicine simply to provide the means to help people accomplish certain ends, irrespective of what those ends are? Without denying that medicine often does that, it has also been assumed that medicine should be governed by an internal ethic that makes it immune from consumer demand. All needs do not count equally. If the aim of medicine is health, then that surely involves moral assumptions about what and how the physician aids patients.

Moreover, even if the problem of "childlessness" is properly understood to be a "medical problem," then why is *in vitro* fertilization assumed to be the most effective therapy? Why do we not instead direct our attention to the development of implantable artificial fallopian tubes? For all I know, we may already have such devices. Indeed, the lack of discussion concerning alternative therapies make one suspicious about whether the purpose of this research is limited to its therapeutic ends. Any intellectual knows the attraction of an "interesting problem." Can we discount that such interests are present in our assumed therapeutic interest in *in vitro* fertilization?

My perspective might be interpreted as but another instance of religious people trying to restrict the progress of science because they fear the consequences. It is certainly true that religious people have often said "no" to science because they are afraid that science will remove the "mystery" of life and thus make religious belief unintelligible. Or they assume that in the absence of any sure way to know God's will, "nature" is our only indication of God's intentions, and to fool with "nature" is thus to disturb God's law. It should be clear, from my remarks, that I do not share this understanding of nature's relation to God; nor do I think that faith in God means assuming that life is finally a "mystery." In contrast, I much prefer to think of life as interesting, an adventure that we can risk because of, and not in spite of, our faith in God. The only mystery the Christian faith has a stake in preserving is the mystery of God's love. All other "mysteries" are but puzzles next to that one.

Rather than treat this again as an issue of religion and science, it should be considered in terms of what ends of community should guide our scientific endeavors. Any conflict between religion and science concerning such matters as *in vitro* fertilization does not lie in the actual technique itself but in the claim that science is autonomous and not subject to guidance or judgment from external authorities. That is indeed a claim that Christians cannot help but challenge. As members of an institution that also claims total loyalty, we recognize other counter-churches. Christians insist that science, practiced morally, must be at the service of community, not its master.

The most important response, however, to the claim that medicine's goal in *in vitro* fertilization is solely to provide individuals with necessary therapy is that such an intention is unjust. For surely the man-hours and resources necessary to develop such a technique are hardly worth the results. This may sound like a harsh judgment to those who want children but are prevented from doing so, but in the classic words of Jimmy Carter, "life is unfair." Surely amid the immense needs of our society, resources can be better spent than developing techniques to allow a very small percentage of women to experience pregnancy. I simply do not understand why that particular problem should be thought so severe that resources should be given to it before we have, for example, a cheap and effective clotting factor for hemophiliacs.

Conclusion

I have not dealt with such issues as the status of the blastocyst,[6] discarded conceptus, how such procedures may produce damaged human beings, or possible misuses of the technique. I have not done so because others have already discussed such matters, but also because I do not think such issues have the same kind of theological interest.

Also, I have not dealt with such matters because they seem to me to direct our attention to the wrong place. For in spite of the theological cast of my argument I hope my position is a call to take seriously what is really at stake in *in vitro* fertilization — namely, common sense.

Of course, as has often been pointed out, nothing is more uncommon than common sense. If we but listen to our common sense I believe we should not fund *in vitro* fertilization, though neither should we as a society prohibit those who wish from pursuing *in vitro* fertilization research. However, in my opinion no Christian should support or engage in such research, as it can only appear to us a pretentious and unjust attempt to substitute biological identity for the moral convictions that should be the substance of familial identity.[7]

NOTES

1. I think it would be extremely interesting to know when the field of "ethics" or the job of the "ethicist" began to be understood as an independent and self-sufficient activity. The Roman Catholic community has "moral theologians" who have had clearly defined tasks correlative to definite institutional needs of the church. But it was not assumed, though it tended to be the practice, that "moral theology" was thereby a coherent or independent intellectual area. In our own context I suspect the idea that "ethics" is an intelligible field is not the result of a coherent intellectual and social position, but results from an attempt of a confused society to substitute thinkers, to create more "experts," for morally substantive convictions.

2. Alasdair MacIntyre [5] has argued forcefully that the dominance of Kantian presuppositions in contemporary moral philosophy has resulted in a failure to acknowledge the intellectual and moral significance of the moral pluralism of our society. In an attempt to provide grounds for moral agreement between people with different beliefs, modern moral philosophy has attempted to make "beliefs" irrelevant to moral judgment, and to make character secondary to moral decisions. As a result moral experience has been distorted, for we are left with insufficient conceptual tools to understand what has happened to us morally. The current emphasis on "rights" as the conceptually primitive or bedrock moral notion is but a further indication of this tendency.

3. For a more extended presentation of this position see [3].

4. For a more extended discussion of this point see [1] and [2].

5. This paragraph and much else in this paper I owe to Anne Harley Hauerwas.

6. Though I do not wish to make much of it, I find the often made claim that blastocyst or conceptus has "some value" to be a conceptual mystification. They obviously want to say that this is human life and thus should be treated with care, i.e., it has "some value," but I fail to understand how something can have "some value." It either has value or it does not. I suspect that the language of "value" cannot provide the kind of discourse needed to understand why we feel hesitant about treating the human conceptus any way we wish for the good ends of science.

7. It might appear that the position I have developed is antithetical to the Jewish understanding of the importance of biological identity for the family. For example, Onan's sin was not (as the Catholics assume) masturbation but his refusal to be open to keeping his brother's name alive in Israel. There is no doubt a stronger emphasis on familial continuity among Jews than among Christians, but for both the "biology" remains secondary to the family understood as a religious and moral institution.

REFERENCE

[1] Hauerwas, Stanley. 1978. "Sex and Politics: Bertrand Russell and 'Human Sexuality.' " *Christian Century* 95, no. 14 (April 19, 1978): 417–422.

[2] Hauerwas, Stanley. 1977. *Truthfulness and Tragedy*. Notre Dame, Ind.: University of Notre Dame Press. See especially pp. 147–163.

[3] Hauerwas, Stanley. 1975. *Character and the Christian Life: A Study in Theological Ethics*. San Antonio: Trinity University Press.

[4] Kass, Leon. 1979. "Ethical Issues in Human *In Vitro* Fertilization, Embryo Culture and Research, and Embryo Transfer." In *HEW Support of Research Involving Human In Vitro Fertilization and Embryo Transfer*, essay no. 2. Washington, D.C.: U.S. Government Printing Office.

[5] MacIntyre, Alasdair. 1984. *After Virtue*. Notre Dame, Ind.: University of Notre Dame Press.

[6] Ramsey, Paul. 1979. "Testimony on *In Vitro* Fertilization," In *HEW Support of Research Involving Human In Vitro Fertilization and Embryo Transfer*, essay no. 7. Washington, D.C.: U.S. Government Printing Office.

[7] Ramsey, Paul. 1970. *Fabricated Man*. New Haven: Yale University Press. See especially pp. 38-39.

[8] Toulmin, Stephen. 1978. "In Vitro Fertilization: Answering Ethical Objections." *Hastings Center Report* 8, no. 5: 9-11.

PART THREE

"Caring" for the Mentally Handicapped

9

Suffering the Retarded:
Should We Prevent Retardation?

A Short Movie and a Question

The movie begins. A man and woman stand looking into a baby crib. The baby is never shown. The room is dark and the countenance of the couple is yet darker. They have obviously been through a trauma and are still in shock. The joy and excitement associated with the birth of a child has been crushed from their lives. Their high expectations have been transformed to absolute despair.

They turn toward us and the man speaks: "Don't let this happen to you. Our child was born retarded. He will never play the way other children play. He will not be able to go to school with other children. He will never have an independent existence and will require us to care for him throughout his and our lifetime. Our lives have been ruined. It is too late for us but not for you."

The mother speaks: "Don't let what happened to us happen to you. Be tested early if you think you are pregnant. Maintain good prenatal care under the direction of a physician. Do not smoke, drink, or take any drugs except those absolutely necessary for your health. Please do not let this happen to you—prevent retardation."

A film very much like this was sponsored a few years ago by the American Association of Retarded Citizens. No doubt the film was made with the best of intentions and concern. Surely we ought to prevent retardation. Certainly as many couples as can ought to be encouraged to maintain good prenatal care. Moreover the Association of Retarded Citizens is probably right to assume they will stand a better chance of getting research funds for the retarded if they can convince the public, and thus the government, that their long-term policy is to eliminate retardation like cancer. For if retardation can be eliminated, then the amount of moneys needed for constant care will

159

be significantly reduced. Better a short-term outlay now than a continuing cost.

Nevertheless there seems to be something deeply wrong, something disturbing about this film and its message, "Prevent Retardation." Perhaps part of the difficulty involves the disanalogy between preventing retardation and preventing cancer, polio, or heart disease, as these latter diseases exist independent of the subjects having diseases. The disease can be eliminated without eliminating the subject of the disease. But the same is not always true of the retarded. To eliminate retardation may sometimes mean to eliminate the subject.

Yet surely this point is not decisive. The film, after all, is not suggesting that we kill anyone who is presently retarded. On the contrary, those who produced the film have dedicated their lives to enhancing of the lives of retarded citizens. They have led the war on unjust forms of discrimination against retarded. They surely do not seek to make the lot of the retarded worse than it is already; rather they simply seek to prevent some from being born unnecessarily retarded. What could be wrong with that?

Still I think something is wrong with a general policy that seeks to prevent retardation, but to say what is wrong with such a policy involves some of the most profound questions of human existence, including our relationship to God. In particular, assumptions about the nature and necessity of suffering, and our willingness to endure it in our own and other's lives, will need to be addressed. For the very humanity that causes us to cry out against suffering, that motivates us to seek to eliminate retardation, is also the source of our potentially greatest inhumanity.

By trying to understand why this is the case, moreover, I hope to illumine how our moral and religious presuppositions shape our medical care. Too often medicine becomes the means by which, in the name of humanity, we eliminate those who suffer. Thus it has become common in our society to assume that certain children born with severe birth defects who also happen to be retarded should not be kept alive in order to spare them a lifetime of suffering. But why do we assume that it is the role of medicine to save us from suffering? By exploring whether we ought to try to eliminate the retarded I hope, therefore, to make explicit a whole set of assumptions about suffering and medicine's role in its alleviation.

Setting the Issues

Before addressing these large issues, however, I think it wise to discern more exactly some of the problems raised by the film as well as some of the problems of the film. It is obvious that the film is in serious conflict with the convictions of many who belong to and support the Association for Retarded Citizens. The film gives the impression that there is nothing more disastrous, nothing more destructive, than for a child to be born retarded, but the sponsoring organization for the film maintains that the retarded are not significantly different from the so-called normal. Indeed, the Association for Retarded Citizens believes that with appropriate training most retarded people can become contributing members of a society even as complex as our own. Thus the negative impression of retardation that the film conveys is not one which those sponsoring the film believe or think warranted. And it could have the unintended effect of reinforcing our society's largely negative attitude toward the retarded.

Perhaps equally troubling is the indiscriminate use of the notion of "retardation" in the film. Not only does the film fail to denote the wide variety of retardation—sometimes much less serious than others—but even more it fails to make clear that our attribution of retardation may be due as much to our prejudices as it is the assumed limits of the retarded. It has become increasingly recognized that disease descriptions and remedies are relative to a society's values and needs. Thus "retardation" might not "exist" in a society which values cooperation more than competition and ambition.

Yet the increasing realization that retardation is a social designation should not blind us to the fact that the retarded do have some quite specifiable problems peculiar to them and that their difference requires special forms of care.

It is extremely important how we put this if we are to avoid two different perils. The first, assuming that societal prejudice is embodied in all designations of retardation, seeks to aid the retarded by preventing discriminatory practices in a manner similar to the civil rights campaigns for blacks and women. Because the retarded are said to have the same rights as anyone, in this view all they require is to be treated "normally." Without denying that the retarded have "rights" or that much good has been done under the banner "normalization," I believe this way of putting the matter is misleading and risks making the retarded subject to even greater societal cruelty.[1] Would it not be unjust to treat the retarded "equally"? Instead, retardation ought to be so precisely understood that those who are thus handicapped can be accommodated as they need.

But that may be a reason for avoiding the word *retardation* altogether. As I have already noted there are so many different ways of being retarded, so many different kinds of disabilities and corresponding forms of care required that to isolate a group as "retarded" may be the source of much of the injustice we perpetrate on those whom we identify as "not normal."

The second peril is that of oppressive care, a kind of care based on the assumption that the retarded are so disabled they must be protected from the dangers and risks of life. Such a strategy subjects the retarded to a cruelty fueled by our sentimental concern to deal with their differences by treating them as something less than human agents. Too often this strategy isolates the retarded from the rest of society in the interest of "protecting" them from societal indifference. As a result they are trained to be retarded.

The challenge is to know how to characterize retardation and to know what difference it should make, without our very characterizations being used as an excuse to treat the retarded unjustly. However, we see this is not just a problem for the retarded, but a basic problem of any society, since societies are only possible because we are all different in skills and different in needs.[2] Societies must find ways to characterize and institutionalize those differences so that we see them as enhancing rather than diminishing each of our lives. From this perspective the retarded are a poignant test of a society's particular understanding of how our differences are relevant to and for achievement of a common good.

The various issues I have raised can be illustrated by pointing to one final fallacy that the film underwrites. It give the impression that retardation is primarily a genetic problem recognized at, or soon after, birth. But that is simply not the case. Half the people who bear the label "retarded" do so as the result of some circumstance after their conception and/or birth. Many are retarded due to environmental, nutritional, and/or accidental causes. To suggest, therefore, that we can eliminate retardation by better prenatal care or more thorough genetic screening and counseling is a mistake. Even if we were all required to have genetic checks before being allowed to marry, we would still have some among us that we currently label as "retarded."

We must ask what the "prevent retardation" campaign would mean for this group? If a society were even partially successful in "eliminating" retardation, how would it regard those who have become retarded? Since retardation was eliminated on grounds of being an unacceptable way of being human, would the retarded who remain live in a society able to recognize the validity of their existence and willing to provide the care they require? Of course it might be suggested that with fewer retarded there would be more resources for the care of those remaining. That is no doubt true, but the question is whether there would be the moral will to direct those resources in their direction. Our present resources are more than enough to provide good care for the retarded. That we do not provide such care can be attributed to a lack of moral will and imagination. What will and imagination there is comes from those who have found themselves unexpectedly committed to care for a retarded person through birth or relation. Remove that and I seriously doubt whether our society will find the moral convictions necessary to sustain our alleged commitment to the retarded.

To reckon whether this is mere speculation, consider this thought experiment. We live at a time when it is possible through genetic screening to predict who has the greatest likelihood of having a retarded child, particularly if that person marries someone of similar genetic characteristics. It has become a general policy for most of the population to have such screening and to choose their marriage partner accordingly. Moreover, amniocentesis has become so routine that the early abortion of handicapped chidren has become the medical "therapy" of choice.

How would such a society regard and treat a couple who refused to be genetically screened, who refused amniocentesis, and who might perhaps have a less than normal child? Would such a society be happy with the increased burden on its social and financial resources? Why should citizens support the birth and care of such a child when its existence could easily have been avoided? To care for such a child, to support such "irresponsible" parents, means only that the "truly" needy will be unjustly deprived of care in the interest of sustaining a child who will never "contribute to societal good." That such an attitude seems not unreasonable to many people also suggests that in our current situation a campaign to "prevent retardation" might have negative implications for those who are retarded, as well as those who may have the misfortune to be born retarded or become retarded in the future.

Suffering and the Retarded

But surely there is something wrong with these observations, as they seem to imply that since we can never ensure that no one will be born or become retarded, then we should not even try to prevent retardation. On such grounds it seems we cannot change our lives to ensure that few will be born retarded so that those who are retarded now and in the future will not be cruelly treated and may even receive better care. That is clearly a vicious and unworthy position. We rightly seek to prevent those forms of retardation that are preventable. To challenge that assumption would be equivalent to questioning our belief that the world is round or that love is a good thing. Like so many things that seem obvious, however, if we ask *why* they seem so, we are often unable to supply an answer. Perhaps they seem obvious precisely because they do not require a reason for holding them.

I suspect that at least part of the reason it seems so obvious that we ought to prevent retardation is the conviction that we ought to prevent suffering. No one should will that an animal should suffer gratuitously. No one should will that a child should endure an illness. No one should will that another person should suffer from hunger. No one should will that a child should be born retarded. That suffering should be avoided is a belief as deep as any we have. That someone born retarded suffers is obvious. Therefore if we believe we ought to prevent suffering, it seems we ought to prevent retardation.

Yet like many other "obvious" beliefs the assumption that suffering should *always* be prevented, if analyzed, becomes increasingly less certain or at least involves unanticipated complexity. Just because it implies eliminating subjects who happen to be retarded should at least suggest to us that something is wrong with our straightforward assumption that suffering should always be avoided or, if possible, eliminated. This is similar to some justifications of suicide: namely, in the interest of avoiding or ending suffering a subject wills no longer to exist. Just because in suicide there is allegedly a decision by the victim does not alter the comparison with some programs to prevent retardation: both assume that certain forms of suffering are so dehumanizing that it is better not to exist.

As I have indicated above, this assumption draws upon some of our most profound moral convictions. Yet I hope to show that our assumption that suffering should *always* be prevented is a serious and misleading oversimplification. To show why this is the case a general analysis of suffering is required. We assume we know what suffering is because it is so common, but on analysis suffering turns out to be an extremely elusive subject. Only once that analysis has been done will we be in a position to ask if the retarded suffer from being retarded or whether the problem is the suffering we feel the retarded cause us.

The Kinds and Ways of Suffering

"To suffer" means to undergo, to be subject. But we undergo much we do not call suffering. Suffering names those aspects of our lives that we undergo and which have a particularly negative sense. We suffer when what we undergo blocks our positive desires and wants. Suffering also carries a sense of "surdness": it denotes those frustrations for which we can give no satisfying explanation and which we cannot make serve some wider end. Suffering thus names a sense of brute power that does violence to our best laid plans. It is not easily domesticated. Therefore, there can be no purely descriptive account of suffering, since every description necessarily entails some judgment about the value or purpose of certain states.

No doubt the intensity of our own suffering or of our sympathy for others' suffering has reinforced our assumptions that we have a firm grip on its meaning. Yet it is certainly not clear that the kind of suffering occasioned by starvation is the same as that of cancer, though each is equally terrifying in its relentless but slow resolution in death. It is interesting that we also use *suffer* in an active sense of "bearing with," permitting, or enduring. While such expressions do not eclipse the passive sense associated with suffering, they at least connote that we do not associate suffering only with that for which we can do nothing.

Perhaps this is the clue we have been needing to understand better the nature of suffering. We must distinguish between those forms of suffering that happen to us and those that we bring on ourselves or that are requisite to our purposes and goals. Some suffering which befalls us is integral to our goals, only we did not previously realize it. We tend to associate pain, however, with that which happens to us, since it seems to involve that which stands as a threat to our goals and projects, rather than as some means to a further end. In like manner, we suffer from illness and accidents — thus our association of pain with sickness and physical trauma. Of course pain and illness are interrelated, because most of the time when we are ill we hurt, but it is also true that conceptually pain and illness seem to stand on that side of suffering that is more a matter of fate than choice.

This distinction helps us to see the wider meaning of suffering. We not only suffer from diseases, accidents, tornadoes, earthquakes, droughts, floods — all those things over which we have little control — but we also suffer from other people, from living here rather than there, from doing this kind of job — all matters we might avoid — because in these instances we see what we suffer as part of a large scheme. This latter sense of "suffer," moreover, seems more subjective, since what may appear as a problem for one may seem an opportunity for another. Not only is what we suffer relative to our projects, but how we suffer is relative to what we have or wish to be.[3]

Without denying the importance of the distinction between forms of suffering that happen to us and those that we instigate as requisite to our goals, we would be mistaken to press it too hard. Once considered, it may not seem as evident or as helpful as it first appeared. For example, we often discuss how what at the time looked like something that happened to us — something we suffered — was in fact something we did, or at least chose not to avoid. Our increasing knowledge of the relation of illness to life-style is enough to make us think twice before drawing a hard and fast distinction between what happens to us and what we do.

But the situation is even more complex. We often find that essential in our response to suffering is the ability to make what happens to me mine. Cancer patients frequently testify to some sense of relief when they find out they have cancer. The very ability to name what they have seems to give them a sense of control or possession that replaces the indifferentiated fear they had been feeling. Pain and suffering alienate us from ourselves. They make us what we do not know. The task is to find the means to make that which is happening to me mine — to interpret its presence (even if such an interpretation is negative) as something I can claim as integral to my indentity. No doubt our power to transform events into decisions can be the source of great self-deception, but it is also the source of our moral identity.

Please note: I am not suggesting that every form of pain or suffering can or should be seen as some good or challenge. Extreme suffering can as easily destroy as enhance. Nor do I suggest that we should be the kind of people who can transform any suffering into benefit. We rightly feel that some forms of suffering can only be acknowledged, not transformed. Indeed, at this point I am not making any normative recommendations about how we should respond to suffering; rather I am suggesting the distinction between the suffering which happens to us and the suffering which we accept as part of our projects is not as clear as it may at first seem. More important is the question of what kind of people we ought to be so that certain forms of suffering are not denied but accepted as part and parcel of our existence as moral agents.

In spite of our inability to provide a single meaning to the notion of suffering or to distinguish clearly between different kinds of suffering, I think this analysis has not been without important implications. It may well be that those forms of suffering we believe we should try to prevent or to eliminate are those that we think impossible to integrate into our projects, socially or individually. It is exactly those forms of suffering which seem to intrude uncontrollably into our lives which appear to be the most urgent candidates for prevention. Thus our sense that we should try to prevent suffering turns out to mean that we should try to prevent those kinds of suffering that we do not feel can serve any human good.

Even this way of putting the matter may be misleading. Some may object that while it is certainly descriptively true that we find it hard to integrate certain kinds of suffering into our individual and social lives, that ought not be the case. The issue is not what we do, but rather who we ought to be in order to be capable of accepting all suffering as a necessary aspect of human existence. In viewing our life narrowly as a matter of purposes and accomplishments, we may miss our actual need for suffering, even apparently purposeless or counterpurposeful suffering. The issue is not whether retarded children can serve a human good, but whether we should be the kind of people, the kind of parents and community, that can receive, even welcome, them into our midst in a manner that allows them to flourish.

But it may be objected that although this latter way of putting the issue seems to embody the highest moral ideals, in fact, it is deeply immoral because the suggestion that all forms of suffering are capable of being given human meaning is destructive of the human project. Certain kinds of suffering—Hiroshima, Auschwitz, wars—are so horrible we are able to preserve our humanity only by denying them human significance. No "meaning" can be derived from the Holocaust except that we must do everything we can to see that it does not happen again. Perhaps individuals can respond to natural disasters such as hurricanes and floods in a positive manner, but humanly we are right to view these other destructions as a scourge which we will neither accept nor try to explain in some positive sense.

Our refusal to accept certain kinds of suffering, or to try to interpret them as serving some human purpose, is essential for our moral health. Otherwise we would far too easily accept the causes of suffering rather than trying to eliminate or avoid them. Our primary business is not to accept suffering, but to escape it, both for our own sake and our neighbor's. Still, in the very attempt to escape suffering, do we not lose something of our own humanity? We rightly try to avoid unnecessary suffering, but it also seems that we are never quite what we should be until we recognize the necessity and inevitability of suffering in our lives.

To be human is to suffer. That sounds wise. That sounds right—that is, true to the facts. But we should not be too quick to affirm it as a norm. Questions remain as to what kind of suffering should be accepted and how it should be integrated into our lives. Moreover, prior to these questions is the even more challenging question of why suffering seems to be our fate. Even if I knew how to answer such questions, I could not try to address them in this paper. (Indeed, I suspect that there can be no general answer that does not mislead as much as it informs.) But perhaps by directing our attention toward the retarded we can better understand why and how suffering is never to be merely "accepted" and yet why it is unavoidable in our lives. In preparation for that discussion, I need to try to suggest why it is that suffering seems so unavoidable.

On Why We Suffer

To ask why we suffer makes the questioner appear either terribly foolish or extremely arrogant. It seems foolish to ask, since in fact we *do* suffer and no sufficient reason can be given to explain that fact. Indeed, if it were explained, suffering would be denied some of its power. The question seems arrogant because it seeks to put us in the position of eating from the tree of good and evil. Only God knows the answer to such questions.

Without denying that the question of why we suffer can be foolish and pretentious, I think it is worth asking since it has one obvious answer: we suffer because we are incomplete beings who depend on one another for our existence. Indeed, the matter can be put more strongly, since we depend upon others not only for our survival but also for our identity. Suffering is built into our condition because it is literally true that we exist only to the extent that we sustain, or "suffer," the existence of others and the others include not just others like us, but mountains, trees, animals, and so on.

This is exactly contrary to cherished assumptions. We believe that our identity derives from our independence, our self-possession. As Arthur McGill suggests, we think "a person is real so far as he can draw a line around certain items — his body, his thoughts, his house — and claim them as his own"([4], p. 89). Thus death becomes our ultimate enemy — the intimation involved in every form of suffering — because it is the ultimate threat to our identity. Again, as McGill suggests, that is why what we suffer so often seems to take proportions: our neediness seems to make us helpless to what we undergo. In this sense, our "neediness represents a fundamental *flaw* in our identity, a basic inability to rest securely with those things which are one's own and which lie inside the line between oneself and the rest of reality. Need forces the self to become open to the not-self; it requires every man to come to terms with the threats of demonic power" ([4], p. 90).

The irony is, however, that our neediness is also the source of our greatest strength, for our need requires the cooperation and love of others from which derives our ability not only to live but to flourish. Our identity, far from deriving from our self-possession, or our self-control, comes from being "de-possessed" of those powers whose promise is only illusory. Believing otherwise, fearful of our sense of need, when we attempt to deny our reliance on others, we become all the more subject to those powers. As we shall see, this has particularly significant implications for our relations with the retarded, since we "naturally" disdain those who do not or cannot cover up their neediness. Prophetlike, the retarded only remind us of the insecurity hidden in our false sense of self-possession.[4]

It may be objected that such an account of suffering is falsely subtle, since it is obvious why we suffer: bad things happen to us. We are injured in accidents; we lose everything in a flood; our community is destroyed by a tornado; we get cancer; a retarded child is born. These are not things that happen to us because of our needs, but rather they happen because they happen. Yet each does relate to concrete needs — the need for security and safety, the need for everydayness, the need for health, the need for new life.[5] If we try to deny any of these needs, as well as many others, we deny ourselves the necessary resources for well-lived lives and make ourselves all the more subject to the powers who draw their strength from our fears.

I have not tried in this brief and inadequate account of why we suffer to offer anything like a theodicy. Indeed, I remain skeptical of all attempts to provide some general account or explanation of evil or suffering. For example, it is by no means clear that evil and suffering raise the same questions, since certainly not every form of suffering is evil. Moreover, as I have suggested above, I do not think any explanation that removes the surdness of certain forms of suffering can be right. Much in our lives should not be made "good" or explained.

All I have tried to do is to state the obvious — we suffer because we are inherently creatures of need. This does not explain, much less justify our suffering or the evil we endure. But it does help us understand why the general policy to prevent suffering is at least odd as a general policy. Our task is to prevent unnecessary suffering, but the hard question, as we have seen, is to know what constitutes unnecessary suffering. It is even more difficult when the question concerns another, as it does in the case of the retarded. It is just that question to which we now must turn.

Do the Retarded Suffer from Being Retarded?

I suggested above that behind the claim that we ought to prevent retardation lies the assumption that we ought to prevent suffering or, in particular, unnecessary suffering. I have tried at least to raise some critical questions about that assumption. But there is another issue that requires equal analysis: Are we right to assume that the retarded are suffering by being retarded? Certainly they suffer retardation, but do they suffer from being retarded?

No doubt, like everyone, the retarded suffer. Like us, they have accidents. Like us, they have colds, sores, and cancer. Like us, they are subject to natural disasters. Like us, they die. But the question is whether they suffer from being retarded. We assume they suffer because of their retardation, just as we or others suffer from being born blind or deaf. Yet it is by no means clear that such cases are similar or even whether those born blind or deaf suffer from blindness or deafness. It is possible that they are in fact taught by us that they are decisively disabled, and thus learn to suffer. If that is the case, then there is at least some difference between being blind and being retarded, since the very nature of being retarded means there is a limit to their understanding of their disadvantage and thus the extent of their suffering. That may also be true of being blind or deaf, of course, but not in the same way.

Do the retarded understand that they are retarded? Certainly most are able to see that they are different than many of us, but there is no reason to think they would on their own come to understand their condition as "retardation" or that they are in some decisive way suffering. They may perceive that there are some things some people do easily which they can do only with great effort or not at all, but that in itself is not sufficient reason to attribute to them great suffering. Of course it may be objected that if we are to care for them, if we are to help alleviate some of the results of their being retarded, we cannot help but try to make them understand their limits. We have to make them conscious of their retardation if we are to help them be free from some of the effects of their condition. But again, this is certainly not as clear as it first appears, for it by no means follows that by learning to confront their limits in order to better their life, the retarded necessarily understand they are thereby suffering from something called "retardation," "Down's Syndrome," or the like.

Yet we persist in the notion that the retarded are suffering and suffering so much from being retarded that it would be better for them not to exist then to have to bear such disability. It is important I not be misunderstood. I am not suggesting that retardation is a minor problem or that nothing should be done to try to prevent, alleviate, or lessen the effects of being retarded; I have tried, rather, to suggest that the widespread assumption that the retarded suffer from being retarded is by no means obviously true.

Perhaps what we assume is not that the retarded suffer from being retarded but rather, because they are retarded, they will suffer from being in a world like ours. They will suffer from inadequate housing, inadequate medical care, inadequate schooling, lack of love and care. They will suffer from discrimination as well as cruel kidding and treatment from unfeeling peers. All this is certainly true, but it is not an argument for preventing retardation in the name of preventing suffering; rather it is an argument for changing the nature of the world in the interest of preventing the needless suffering we impose on the retarded.

It may be observed that we have very little hope that the world will or can be changed in this respect, but even if that is the case it would be insufficient grounds for the general policy of eliminating the retarded. On such grounds anyone suffering injustice or ill-treatment would be in jeopardy. If justice comes to mean the elimination of the victim of injustice rather than the cause of injustice, we stand the risk of creating admittedly a less troubled but deeply unjust world.

The need to subject this set of assumptions to rigorous analysis is particularly pressing in relation to the care of children born retarded or otherwise handicapped. A policy of nontreatment is often justified as a means of sparing a child a life of suffering. I by no means wish to argue that every child should receive the most energetic medical care to keep it alive, but if such care is withheld it cannot be simply to spare the child a life of suffering. On such grounds few children with any moderately serious chronic health problem would be cared for at birth. We all, healthy and nonhealthy, normal or abnormal, are destined for a life of suffering.

Some will say that this is surely to miss the point behind the concern to spare certain children a life of suffering. The issue is the extent and intensity of the suffering. But again such a judgment is a projection of our assumptions about how we would feel if we were in their situation. But that is exactly what we are not. We do not know to what extent they may suffer from their disability. We do not know how much pain they will undergo, but we nonetheless act to justify our lack of care in the name of our humane concern about their destiny. We do so even knowing that our greatest nobility as humans often derives from the individual's struggle to make positive use of his or her limitations.

I am not suggesting that the care we give to severely disabled children (or adults) will always result in happy results for themselves or those around them. But to refrain from such care to spare them future suffering can be a formula for profound self-deception. Too often the suffering we wish to spare them is the result of our unwillingness to change our lives so that those disabled might have a better life. Or, even more troubling, we refrain from life-giving care simply because we do not like to have those who are different from us to care for.

Our Suffering of the Retarded

Why, therefore, do we persist in assumptions that the retarded suffer from being retarded? At least something of an answer comes from a most unlikely source: Adam Smith's *Theory of Moral Sentiments*. In that book Smith endeavors to provide an account for why, no matter how "selfish a man may be supposed, there are evidently some principles in his nature which interest him in the fortune of others, and render their happiness necessary to him, though he derives nothing from it except the pleasure of seeing it" ([7], p.1, 1). Such a sentiment, Smith observes, is by no means confined to the virtuous, since even the most "hardened ruffian" at times may derive sorrow from the sorrow of others.

Still, according to Smith, this is something of a puzzle. Since we have no "immediate experience of what other men feel, we can form no idea of the manner in which they are affected, but by conceiving what we ourselves should feel in the like situation. Though our brother is upon the rack, as long as we ourselves are at our ease, our senses will never inform us what he suffers. They never did, and never can, carry us beyond our own person, and it is by the imagination only that we can form any conception of what are his sensations" ([7], p. 1, 2).

It is through our imagination, therefore, that our fellow-feeling with the sorrow of others is generated. But our sympathy does not extend to every passion, for there are some passions that disgust us—thus the furious behavior of an angry man may actually make us more sympathetic with his enemies. That this is so makes us especially anxious to be people capable of eliciting sympathy from others. Thus "sympathy enlivens joy and alleviates grief. It enlivens joy by presenting another source of satisfaction; and it alleviates grief by insinuating unto the heart almost the only agreeable sensation which it is at that time capable of receiving" ([7], p. 1, 1). By knowing our sorrow is shared by another we seem to be less burdened with our distress. Moreover, we are pleased when we are able to sympathize with one who is suffering, but we look forward more to enjoying another's good fortune.

Because we seek to sympathize as well as be the object of sympathy, Smith observes:

> Of all the calamities to which the condition of mortality exposes mankind, the loss of reason appears, to those who have the least spark of humanity, by far the most dreadful, and they behold that last stage of human "wretchedness" with deeper commiseration than any other. But the poor wretch, who is in it, laughs and sings perhaps, and is altogether insensible of his own misery. The anguish which humanity feels, therefore, at the sight of such an object, cannot be the reflection of any sentiment of the sufferer. The compassion of the spectator must arise altogether from the consideration of what he himself would feel if he was reduced to the same unhappy situation, and, what perhaps is impossible, was at the same time able to regard it with his present reason and judgment. ([7], p. 1, 11)

We thus persist in our assumption that the retarded suffer from being retarded not because we are unsympathetic with them but because we are not sure how to be sympathetic with them. We fear that the very imagination which is the source of our sympathy, on which our fellow-feeling is founded, is not shared by them. To lack such an important resource, we suspect, means they are fatally flawed, for one thus lacks the ability to be the subject of sympathy. We seek to prevent retardation not because we are inhumane but because we fear the retarded lack the means of giving and receiving sympathy, and thus we cannot imagine how they feel. Exactly because we are unsure they have the capacity to suffer as we suffer, we seek to avoid their presence in order to avoid the limits of our own sympathy.

As Smith observes, we have no way to know what the retarded suffer as retarded. All we know is how we imagine we would feel if we were retarded. We thus often think we would rather not exist at all than to exist as one retarded. As a result, we miss the point at issue. For the retarded do not feel or understand their retardation as we do, or imagine we would, but rather as they do. We have no right or basis to attribute our assumed unhappiness or suffering to them.

Ironically, therefore, the policy of preventing suffering is one based on a failure of imagination. Unable to see like the retarded, to hear like the retarded, we attribute to them our suffering. We thus rob them of the opportunity to do what each of us must do—learn to bear and live with our individual sufferings.

Need, Loneliness, and the Retarded

In many respects, however, our inability to sympathize with the retarded—to see their life as they see it, to suffer their suffering—is but an aspect of a more general problem. As Smith observes, we do not readily expose our sufferings, because none of us are anxious to identify with the sufferings of others. We try to present a pleasant appearance in order to elicit fellow-feeling with others. We fear to be sufferers, to be in pain, to be unpleasant, because we fear so desperately the loss of fellow-feeling on the part of others. We resent those who suffer without apology, as we expect the sufferer at least to show shame in exchange for our sympathy.

As much as we fear suffering, we fear more the loneliness that accompanies it. We try to deny our neediness as much, if not more so, to ourselves as to others. We seek to be strong. We seek to be self-possessed. We seek to deny that we depend on others for our existence. We will be self-reliant and we resent and avoid those who do not seek to be like us—the strong. We will be friends to one another only so long as we promise not to impose seriously our sufferings on the others. Of course, we willingly enter into some of our friends' suffering—indeed to do so only reinforces our sense of strength—but we expect such suffering to be bounded by a more determinative strength.

That we avoid the sufferer is not because we are deeply unsympathetic or inhumane, but because of the very character of suffering. By its very nature suffering alienates us not only from one another but from ourselves, especially suffering which we undergo, which is not easily integrated into our ongoing projects or hopes. To suffer is to have our identity threatened physically, psychologically, and morally. Thus our suffering even makes us unsure of who we are.

It is not surprising, therefore, that we should have trouble with the suffering of others. None of us willingly seeks to enter into the loneliness of others. We fear such loneliness may result in loss of control of our own life. We feel we must be very strong to be able to help the weak and needy. We may be right about that, but we may also fail to understand the kind of help they really need. Too often we seek to do something rather than first simply learn how to be with, to be present to, the sufferer in his or her loneliness. We especially fear, if not dislike, those whose suffering is the kind for which we can do nothing.

The retarded, therefore, are particularly troubling for us. Even if they do not suffer by being retarded, they are certainly people in need. Even worse, they do not try to hide their needs. They are not self-sufficient, they are not self-possessed, they are in need. Even more, they do not evidence the proper shame for being so. They simply assume that they are what they are and they need to provide no justification for being such. It is almost as if they have been given a natural grace to be free from the regret most of us feel for our neediness.

That such is the case, however, does not mean that the retarded do not suffer from the general tendency of wanting to be self-sufficient. Like us they are more than capable of engaging in the self-deceptive project of being their own person. Nor is such an attempt entirely wrong, for they, like us, rightly seek to develop skills that can help them help themselves as well as others. yet we perceive them as essentially different from us, as beings whose condition has doomed them to a loneliness we fear worse than suffering itself, and, as a result, we seek to prevent retardation.

That we are led to such an extreme derives partly from our frustration at not being able to cure the retarded. We seek to help them overcome their disability, but we know that even our best efforts will not result in the retarded not being retarded. After all, what we finally seek is not simply to help the retarded better negotiate their disability but to be like us: not retarded. Our inability to accomplish that frustrates and angers us, and sometimes the retarded themselves become the object of our anger. We do not like to be reminded of the limits of our power, and we do not like those who remind us.

We fervently seek to help the retarded, to do for the retarded, to make their lot less subject to suffering. No doubt much good derives from such efforts. But our frenzied activity can also be a failure to recognize that our attempts to help, our attempt "to do for" the retarded must first be governed by our ability to be "with" the retarded. Only as we learn to be and do with the retarded, do we learn that their retardation, our projection of their suffering, need not create an unbridgeable gap between them and us. We learn that they are not incapable of fellow-feeling with us and, just as important, that we are not incapable of fellow-feeling with them.

That such fellow-feeling is possible does not mean that they are "really just like us. " They are not. They do not have the same joys we have nor do they suffer just as we suffer. But in our joys and in our sufferings they recognize something of their joy and their suffering, and they offer to share their neediness with us. Such an offer enables us in quite surprising ways to discover that we have needs to share with them. We are thus freed from the false and vicious circle of having to appear strong before others' weakness, and we are then able to join with the retarded in the common project of sharing our needs and satisfactions. As a result we discover we no longer fear them.

I am not suggesting that such sharing comes easily. Few of us are prepared to enter naturally into such a life. Indeed most of us, cherishing the illusion of our strength, must be drawn in reluctantly. But miraculously many are so graced. Day in and day out, through life with their retarded child, brother, or friend, they learn to see themselves through the eyes of the other who happens also to be retarded. Moreover, by learning not to fear the other's retardation, they learn not to fear their own neediness.

Thus if we are to make a movie to help others avoid unnecessary risks that can result in retardation, let us not begin soon after the birth. To begin there is grossly unfair, because it catches us before we are even sure what has happened to us. Let the film begin several years after the birth, after the parents of a child born retarded have discovered, like all parents must, that they are capable of dealing with this. It is not the child they would have willed, but then all children turn out to be different than our expectations. This child, to be sure, raises particular challenges, but let the film show the confidence of the couple that comes from facing those challenges. Unless suggestions for avoiding retarded children are bounded by such confidence, we cannot help but make the life of the retarded that much more difficult. But even more destructive, such a campaign is bound to make our own illusory fears of the retarded and our own needs that much more powerful.

An Inconclusive Theological Postscript

It may well be asked what all this has to do with our religious convictions as Christians. Of course some obvious connections can be drawn. Christians are alleged to be concerned with the weak and the downtrodden. The retarded seem to fit that description. Since the position developed generally supports the ideal of help for the retarded, it seems consistent with such a religious sentiment.

Or it may be suggested that Christians are a people who have learned to accept that life is under God's direction. They attribute to God the bad as well as the good. Parents, in particular, think it presumptuous to try to determine the quality of their offspring. They accept their retarded, as well as their more nearly normal children, as God's will. They do not presume arrogantly to ask why, or to what purpose, retarded children are born.

There is some truth to each of these positions, but they have to be stated much more carefully. Concern with the downtrodden can too easily result in sentimental acceptance and care of the retarded that fails to respect the integrity of their existence. It condemns the retarded to being "weak" so that they might receive our "charity" rather than acknowledging them to be essential members of our community. The second position, God's will, has been and is used wrongly to justify acceptance of avoidable suffering and injustice.

Yet these more obvious theological connections are not the most significant for helping us understand how we as Christians should respond to the retarded. Quite simply, the challenge of learning to know, to be with, and care for the retarded is nothing less than learning to know, be with, and love God. God's face is the face of the retarded; God's body is the body of the retarded; God's being is that of the retarded. For the God we Christians must learn to worship is not a god of self-sufficient power, a god who in self-possession needs no one; rather ours is a God who needs a people, who needs a son. Absoluteness of being or power is not a work of the God we have come to know through the cross of Christ ([4], p. 75).

Arthur McGill has perceptively interpreted the classical trinitarian debate in this fashion. He suggests:

> The issue between Arius and Athansius has nothing to do with whether God is one or two or three. It has to do with what quality makes God divine, what quality constitutes his perfection. From the perspective of self-contained absoluteness and transcendent supremacy, Arius can only look upon God's begetting a Son as grotesque blasphemy. God, he observed, must be very imperfect if he must generate a Son in order

to become complete. But from the perspective of self-communicating love, Athanasius can look upon the dependent derived Son, not as a blot upon God's divinity, but as a mode of its perfection. Love and not transcendence, giving and not being superior, are qualities that mark God's divinity. Since giving entails receiving, there must be a receptive, dependent, needy pole within the being of God. It is pride — and not love — that fears dependence and that worships transcendence. ([4], p. 78)

That is why in the face of the retarded we are offered an opportunity to see God, for like God they offer us an opportunity of recognizing the character of our neediness. In truth the retarded in this respect are but an instance of the capacity we each have for one another. That the retarded are singled out is only an indication of how they can serve for us all as a prophetic sign of our true nature as creatures destined to need God and, thus, one another.

Moreover, it is through such a recognition that we learn how God would have the world governed. As we are told in the Epistle to Diognetus in answer to the question of why God sent his Son: "to rule as a tyrant, to inspire terror and astonishment? No, he did not. No, he sent him in gentleness and mildness. To be sure, as a king sending his royal son, he sent him as God. But he sent him as to men, as saving and persuading them, and not as exercising force. For force is no attribute to God" ([4], p. 82). But if force is no attribute of God's governance, suffering is. Unlike us, God is not separated from himself or us by his suffering; rather, his suffering makes it possible for him to share our life and for us to share his.

Learning to share our life with God is no doubt difficult — it must be at least as demanding as learning that we can share life with the retarded. But that such a sharing of our sufferings as well as our joys is necessary cannot be doubted. For a world where there is no unpatterned, unpurposeful suffering would be devoid of the means for us to grow out of our selfishness and into love. That is why those who worship such a God are obligated to be confident that we can live well with those whose difference from ourselves we have learned to characterize by the unfortunate label "retarded." For if we did not so learn to live, we know we would be decisively retarded: retarded in our ability to turn ourselves to other's needs, regardless of the cost.[6]

NOTES

1. For an excellent critique of the use of "rights" language in relation to retardation see [3].

2. See for example [2].

3. The relation between suffering and luck certainly would be fruitful to explore. Like suffering, luck involves aspects of life over which we have no control, yet we persist in thinking some forms of good and bad luck are "deserved." The latter judgment seems to imply that someone has "tempted fate" and thus got what he or she deserved. We, therefore, tend to assume that certain kinds of suffering, like certain form of luck, go with particular forms of life. For extremely interesting discussions of luck see [5] and [8].

4. This sense of the prophetic character of the retarded I learned from Dr. Bonita Raine. See in particular [6].

5. I suspect this is one of the reasons the ARC film appeals to parents, for all parents are frustrated by the presence of a retarded child. Most parents suffer willingly for their children if they think such suffering will make their children "better." The problem with the retarded is they seem to offer little hope of ever being decisively better. So we are tempted to eliminate retarded children because of our unwillingness to suffer for a child who will never get better. Of course parents of retarded children soon learn, as finally all parents of normal children also learn, that they can rejoice in their children's "progress" even if such progress fails to correspond to their original ambitions for their children's "betterment."

6. Much in this paragraph I have learned from Rev. James Burtchaell. I also need to thank Mr. Phil Foubert, Rev. Paul Wadell, and Dr. Bonita Raine for reading and criticizing an earlier draft of this article and making valuable suggestions for its improvement.

REFERENCES

[1] Hauerwas, Stanley. 1979. "Reflections on Suffering, Death, and Medicine," *Ethics in Science and Medicine* 6: 229–237. Reprinted in the present volume (see essay no. 1).

[2] Hauerwas, Stanley. 1977. "Community and Diversity: The Tyranny of Normality," *National Apostolate for the Mentally Retarded* 8, 1-2, pp. 20–22. Reprinted in the present volume (see essay no. 12).

[3] Hoffmaster, Barry. 1982. "Caring for Retarded Persons: Ideals and Practical Choices." In Stanley Hauerwas, ed., *Responsibility for Devalued Persons: Ethical Interactions between Society, the Family, and the Retarded*, 24–38. Springfield, Ill.: Charles Thomas Press.

[4] McGill, Arthur. 1983. *Suffering: A Test Case of Theological Method*, Philadelphia: Westminster Press.

[5] Nagel, Thomas. 1979. *Mortal Questions*. Cambridge: Cambridge University Press. See especially pp. 24–38.

[6] Raine, Bonita. 1982. "Care and Mentally Retarded People: Pastoral Dimensions Appropriate to Christian Ethical Convictions." Dissertation, University of Notre Dame.

[7] Smith, Adam. 1976. *The Theory of Moral Sentiments*, ed. D. D. Raphael and A. L. Macfie. Oxford: Oxford University Press.

[8] Williams, Bernard. 1981. *Moral Luck*. Cambridge: Cambridge University Press.

10

The Moral Challenge of the Handicapped

with Bonita Raine

Ethical questions related to how and wherein we care for handicapped people find their answers rooted deeply in our understanding of the place children have in the lives of our communities, the nature of those communities, and how we as community members are willing to recognize and respect those different from us. The readiness of our ecclesial communities to address the challenge of acceptance and welcome is perhaps even more significant than it is for our non-Christian counterparts. Handicapped people in general, and retarded people in particular, live under a special burden in our society. It is as if they bear the burden of proof for living at all or for justifying the care they might receive. Parents of handicapped children can report example after example of how they have had to struggle to secure even the most minimal of care for their children.

Sadly, ecclesial communities within the Christian tradition have done little by explicit teaching or example to counter this trend in a wider society. While ethical imperatives of the Gospel seem clear and have never been forgotten by our churches, the direction which they might offer us as community members has not surfaced as a compelling rationale for caring for our handicapped members or for cherishing as an achievable ideal their total integration into our community. While it is indisputable that Christians through the ages have sought to serve their retarded brethren in some manner or other, there has never been a cohesive or explicit moral notion as to how they should be cared for or how aggressively we should address the issue of their presence among us.

Why is this the case? What makes being retarded such a disability as to exclude them from our secular and ecclesial communities? Are handicapped people not born like any of us with limits and possibilities? Why do the particular limits which we classify as "handicapping conditions" seem to relegate them to the category of last helped and first ignored? Is it because they simply lack the skills which are particularly important in a technologically complex society such as ours? Is the problem that they lack the means to negotiate any society? Or is the problem more properly situated in our communities: do we lack the moral resources to integrate into our communities those whom we perceive to be particularly different from the rest of us?

We cannot hope in this short article to answer all these questions, but we hope at least to suggest the moral challenge that retarded people present us with. It should be said at the outset that we write not as disinterested observers, but as people committed to the care and well-being of retarded people. But we are well aware that such commitment needs defense if we are to make an effective case for why it is so morally important that our communities be willing to have handicapped people among us. As theologians, we propose to explore resources from which we in the Christian community can draw moral arguments to support such a commitment to the presence of our handicapped members.

Of course, it has not always been the case that we have allowed handicapped people to be present in our communities. No matter how inadequate our treatment of retarded people may now be, no matter how ineffectual some of the institutions we relegate them to are, no matter how insufficient state funding may be for essential services, we can comfort ourselves that at least we no longer kill them or "let them die." But before we congratulate ourselves too much for that, we should think again about our treatment of retarded people. For even if we do not kill them, and there are indications that our society may well be rethinking its restraint in that respect, we often come as close as we can while still maintaining the illusion that we are a good and humane society.

Models of custodial or quasi-institutional care to which we relegate retarded children for "training" and "education" provide us with exhibit one. The very idea of "retardation" is often one way we have of labeling and thus of denying status to children born with certain disabilities that scare and bother us. In fact we do not even know what "retardation" means or whether it is a meaningful category. Experts fight over such distinctions as profound, severe, or moderate retardation, but often the reality of the retarded person gets lost entirely in the maze of purported diagnoses or prognoses for educational achievement. What we do not want to admit is that the very label "retardation" tells us more about who *we* are than it does about handicapped people. For "retardation" is but a designation that indicates that certain people cannot perform certain skills at a particular age, but why does that put them morally at a disadvantage? Because our society stresses the importance of intelligence and the power it gives us to take control over our lives, those who appear to be powerless lack value and esteem in our communities. But should we not equally value other human powers, such as the ability to respond to others with love and gratitude? And why should these human powers not assume even greater authority within our ecclesial communities?

Perhaps that is why the retarded scare us so much — namely, they remind us that for all our pretension we are as helpless as they are when all is said and done. Like them, we depend on others for our lives and for the simple things that make life liveable. We prefer to keep our dependence hidden, however, as we are under the illusion that, unlike the retarded, we are in control of our existence. Thus we label those who are so clearly dependent as "retarded" in order to mark them off from us. To Christians, such a distinction must be particularly anathema, for the very content of revelation is to teach us precisely that we are indeed a dependent people.

Therefore morally one of the first important things to recognize when dealing with retarded people is that the very way we are taught to perceive and relate to them is an ethic. To begin our reflection by asking, "How ought we to treat the retarded?" is already too late, as it presupposes that the category retardation makes sense. But to be retarded is not finally a scientific or medical description, it is a moral claim that puts some people at a disadvantage simply because they seem different from most of us in humanly significant ways.

Thus, one of the first and most important ethical strategies for dealing with retarded people is to make sure we get to know them. Our fears are all the more intense the more they are based on ignorance. Often we fear retarded people, and handicapped people generally, because we do not know them. Thus, all we can think about is that "I would rather be dead than be retarded" and, as a result, we fail to appreciate what it might feel like to be retarded. While retarded people do not have the same resources to perceive the environment in the same way as those of us who are not retarded, they feel and act on the world in their own way, which should be no less valued or esteemed than what we claim is the norm.

But, of course, this raises profound moral questions which our society seems to have inadequate resources to deal with. For it is true that retarded people are different—though their differences vary greatly from one individual to another. The question is how we are rightfully to characterize their differences without that very characterization working to undermine their status as full and contributing members of the human and, in particular, Christian community.

It is certainly true, for example, that retarded people need help in developing particular kinds of skills that may come more easily to others. But it seems almost impossible to institute programs for the development of those skills without at the same time ghettoizing the retarded into "special education" or "special services" programs. As a result, we continue to underwrite the isolation that we have seen is already part of the problem. We have no intention of entering the complex, confusing, and controversial issue of "mainstreaming," but it is a graphic illustration of our dilemma. Retarded people cannot justly be treated "just like anyone else," as they often do require "special education" which allows them to develop skills to interact in society in culturally normative ways. At the same time, to the extent they are singled out for "special" treatment, we reinforce the unjust characterization of what it means to be retarded.

This kind of dilemma only indicates why ethically the challenge that retarded people present is much more profound than is usually presumed. It is not simply a matter of coming out with ethical principles that can justify better and more extensive treatment of the retarded; it is not simply a matter of trying to suggest those values that are inherent in all life that underwrite claims of the dignity of the retarded. Rather, the true moral question is what kind of community ought we to be so that we can welcome and care for the other in our midst without that "otherness" being used to justify discrimination?

While this question is raised in a peculiarly intense way by the presence of the retarded, it is but part of the larger question of the place of children in our lives. We live in a society which is unsure why and what value having children entails. People have children because they are fun, or to complement their personalities, or because they do not want to be lonely, and so on—all reasons that the reality of children finally challenge. Thus our society increasingly tolerates children only as potential adults. We put up with their "childness" only because we think it will soon be over and they will be like us.

Of course, there is certain appropriateness to that, as it is the task of any community to intitiate children into an adult world, a world that should enhance their increasing maturity. The problem, however, is when implications of that process seem to mean that there is something wrong with being a child. What needs to be said is that there is nothing wrong with being a child when we are children, but we grow up and rightfully need to change. But, when we think we need to say that there is something wrong with being a child to justify the child's initiation into the adult world, we put the retarded person at a serious disadvantage. For that "adult world" is often one with characteristics that retarded people can never enter—especially as it is associated with learning to stand on your own two feet—and thus the retarded are condemned to be treated as eternal children. If they demand, as they do, to be treated differently, our society feels betrayed, as the assumption is that all the special care they receive can be justified only because they are eternal children.

Every parent and person who knows or works with retarded people knows well this cruel dilemma. For our very concern to care and protect retarded people can so easily become a way to deny them power to determine their own lives. Thus, morally, nothing is more destructive than the solicitous kind of care that tries to protect them from the kind of mistakes we all make and the consequences they and we must therefore suffer. This problem is only made worse when it is transmitted at the social policy level so that retarded people are only given "help" as long as they continue to act as we think retarded people should.

We have tried in this short essay to locate what we take to be some of the central ethical challenges raised by the presence of retarded people in our lives. We have not tried to provide any "solutions" to these challenges. But, from our convictions which come from deep within the Christian tradition, we have tried to suggest the fundamental concern that must be met if we are to work toward a solution—namely, that we must be that kind of people who are capable of recognizing the other without fear and/or resentment. If we can be this kind of community, then we may find that we do not even need the label "retarded," and that we can explore more creative ways at once to help those different from us without that help becoming a form of discrimination.

It is just such a community that the American National Conference of Catholic Bishops called us to be in their "Pastoral Statement on the Handicapped" issued in November 1978. While Catholic authorities have in the past issued generic statements concerning the value of oppressed, downtrodden, and disadvantaged peoples generally, this is the first major document setting forth explicit pastoral guidelines for addressing the dilemmas which handicapped people face, both in our society and in our ecclesial communities. The bishops candidly acknowledge that the church's ministry to handicapped people has been sporadic and too often only at the urging of public opinion or circumstances, presumably from outside the church.

Such an admission follows the bishops' reflections on the nature of prejudice and its relationship to perceptions of difference. It is not coincidental, we believe, that this observation about the church's activity is linked to the notion that "we tend all too often to think of them as somehow apart — not fully 'one of us.' " Our concerns about the nature of community, especially ecclesial community, are also addressed by the bishops. While they affirm Christians' obligation to seek with handicapped people justice in a wider society, the bishops suggest what it is the church should be if it is to retain fidelity to the task to which Christ called it. They suggest that the notion of interdependence is critical and that openness to discovery in diversity or difference is vital. Such a community, they say, will actively work to make the rights of handicapped people real in the fabric of modern society. The bishops are nowhere more eloquent, however, than when they describe the warm acceptance with which handicapped people should be gratefully welcomed in the ecclesial community wherein we can all benefit from their spiritual gifts and the self-realization they share with the rest of us in the Christian community, namely, that "we all live in the shadow of the cross." That shadow reminds us that we are all "marginal" people, and hence our need for mutual integration.

Some may think that our views and those of the Catholic bishops in this respect are nothing short of utopian. While it is true that the wider society is not such a community, it is barely true that such community exists within our churches. We continue to fear that we are destined to live in a world which cannot get along without a label such as "retarded" or "handicapped" in order to domesticate our fear of the other. Ethically, we cannot and should not avoid the struggles which we will have year in and year out, both in the wider society and in our ecclesial communities, to advocate even the most basic care for our retarded members. But neither should we be under the misperception that this is the primary "ethical" issue raised by the retarded.

Rather, we must recognize that those people who call themselves Christians, who claim that they have no fear of the other exactly because they worship a God who is as other as any retarded person, have peculiar moral resources to receive retarded people into their community. In such a community, perhaps help can be extended to people without that help being an occasion for exerting power over their lives. Perhaps in such a community, because it values people not for the power they command, retarded people can be appreciated as inherently valuable.

11

The Retarded, Society, and the Family: The Dilemma of Care

The Retarded and the Family: Our Unexamined Assumptions

It is a commonplace that the family, in particular the family of retarded children, should have the primary responsibility for the care of their children. This is not simply because parents, due to their proximity, are assumed to know best what their children need. Rather, our society's commitment to care physically and morally for children through the agency of their parents is based on the profound assumption that the family has or should have moral priority over all other institutions and values. Thus, Gliedman and Roth, in their book *The Unexpected Minority*, argue that

> the parent's rights over the child take precedence over the professional's personal moral views. To put it bluntly, the professional exists to further the parent's vision of the handicapped child's future. Should the professional disagree, he has every right to try to *persuade* the parent to adopt a different view. He also has every right to give advice when the parent is confused and seeks guidance and emotional support. But except in the most extreme instances of parental incompetence and brutality, such as child abuse, the professional has no right to use his immense moral and practical power to intimidate or to manipulate the parent.[1]

The fact that parents are often manipulated, if not bullied, by professionals does not mean that the primacy of the family is not a working norm for our society. Indeed we can and do criticize the tendency toward professional dominance exactly because of our deep and profound adherence to the family as the locus of moral and physical support for children. Parents have the right to make decisions that will affect their children's lives because we assume that parents are, or should be, the best representatives of their children's interest.

189

However, like most commonplaces, our assumption about our commitment to the family is seldom made explicit, much less subjected to rigorous analysis. Why do we think the family should have such high moral status or why should parents make the basic decisions concerning the care of their children? For example, why do we support the presumption that simply because a man and a woman are able to conceive a child they should be the ones to raise and determine what should or should not be done for that child? Biological identity certainly is not sufficient to make one a parent, for we view "being a parent" as fundamentally a moral role with definite tasks and privileges.

Exactly what that moral competency involves is not a matter we subject to rigorous investigation; rather, we tend to assume that if a couple is capable of producing a child they probably also have the "maturity" to know how to care for and raise children. We assume this even though we are increasingly aware that this is simply not the case. The problem of teenage pregnancy is but the tip of the iceberg, as many people who have children lack any sense whatsoever of the moral skills required for becoming a parent.

It is important to note that the question is not whether parents have the material resources necessary to have children, but whether they have the moral resources for such a task. For the priority of the family for the care and nurture of children is primarily a moral commitment that need not, though it often does, imply the presence of economic means to provide that care. We might well think some families, such as those who have retarded children, should receive material support from elsewhere without qualifying our assumption that the family is morally primary. However, in our kind of society, it is hard to maintain the independence of such a moral commitment where equal financial independence is lacking. The rule still pertains that where the queen's shilling appears, the queen is not far behind.

The fact that we do not subject to rigorous analysis our assumption of the primacy of the family for the care of children is not simply due to intellectual obstinacy. Rather, our willingness to allow anyone capable of conceiving children to do so is based on our profound commitment to individual freedom. In the name of individual rights, we refrain as a society from interfering with a couple's decision to have children, no matter how incompetent we think they might be. Moreover, in the name of protecting the "sacredness" of the family, we also refrain from trying to determine how parents should care for their children.[2]

In the process, we fail to notice that the appeal to "freedom" or "rights" of people to be parents distorts the traditional basis for the moral primacy of the family. Traditionally, parents were assumed to have overriding responsibility for their children because they were assumed capable and could be held accountable for performing certain duties. For example, the family was granted priority to the state in matters dealing with education of children because it was assumed that the family had the responsibility to transmit the wisdom of our culture. Presently, however, appeals to these substantive responsibilities seem to qualify the freedom of the individual, especially if they are in any way used to set social policy involving the having and raising of children. We think we have a right to become a parent irrespective of the kind of person and thus parent we may be or become.

Moreover, I suspect most of us feel no great need to analyze or make explicit the moral presumptions surrounding parenthood, because we think we know what we are doing when we become parents. We have children because we assume that it will be a rewarding experience both for them and for us. We look forward to having children, assuming that the business of raising children is a normal task that requires no extraordinary moral or intellectual skills. Almost anyone can do it, though there may be a few rocky moments for even the best prepared.

I suspect that one of the reasons the discovery that our child is retarded comes as such a shock and jolt is that our assumptions about why we have children have seemed too obvious to examine. After all, this is not what we counted on and certainly does not seem part of the implicit agreement that we assumed we were making in our decision to have a child. We were willing to devote large resources of time, energy, and money for the rearing of this child on the assumption that we would be dealing with a fairly normal being. To have to raise and care for a retarded child simply seems unfair, given our assumptions about having a child in the first place. All those plans for camping trips, football games, or intellectual sharing of ideas too quickly die in the struggle to attain the minimal skills. Suddenly, rather than learning to read by three, we are rejoicing at learning bladder control by twelve.

That such is the case I think also accounts for the reaction of parents of normal children to parents of retarded children. The former do not like to get too close to the latter, since their very presence is a reminder that none of us are very sure what we are doing when we become parents. Parents of retarded children soon discover that most of their relations with other adults, outside the work place, involve those who also have retarded children. Parents of retarded children are often regarded with a great deal of suspicion by parents of normal children as the latter suspect that the extraordinary time and energy put into caring for these children — time that rarely seems worth it, given the level of accomplishment — is really but a way of trying to assuage guilt for having had the bad luck of having a retarded child in the first place.

We thus prefer to keep the retarded and their parents at arm's length, because their presence raises a question most of us prefer remain unasked — namely, what commitments are involved in being a parent that seem to require that we care for these children? We assume that our commitment to the family as the locus of care for children is sufficient to answer this question; however, I have tried to suggest that our inability to spell out what is involved morally in being a parent makes that an extremely ambiguous undertaking. I will try to show that it is not enough to assume parents ought to care for their children, retarded and nonretarded, for that assumption simply is not sufficient to inform us about what kind of care parents should provide. Unless we know more about the kind of care parents should provide, then the commitment of parents to their children loses its moral intelligibility. Indeed, unless these additional aspects of the moral claims implicated in parenting are made explicit, appeals to the priority of the family for the care of children can have the ironic effect of leaving us morally groundless and defenseless in cases when the care provided for the child is literally destructive.

The Priority of the Family: The Example of Parents of the Retarded

I am not going to try to provide a theory for why we think the family should have priority in caring for children. Nor am I going to appeal to any abstract principles to try to suggest the kind of responsibilities that we have as parents for our children. What we must admit is that our culture simply lacks any consensus sufficient to provide a satisfactory response to either of these questions.[3] Rather, I want to draw our attention to what parents of retarded children do, even if they often are unable to say why it is they do what they do. For it is my contention that they have more to teach us than anyone about why we are right in thinking that the family is and should be the primary locus for care of children, both normal and retarded.

I think this way of proceeding is partly justified by the obvious fact that most of us learn what it means to be a parent from our children. Their needs teach us our responsibilities. We simply learn to be a parent through the thousands of small things that we learn to do on a day-to-day basis to meet the demands of sustaining and raising our children. However, we must still learn to say what it is that we have learned. (Indeed, one of the primary reasons inhibiting many from becoming parents today involves our inability to pass the skills of parenting from one generation to another. For parenting is not a "natural" role, but involves skills that can be acquired only by learning them from others. Unfortunately, we seem to lack people who have confidence that they possess those skills to the degree that they are capable of handing them on to us.)

The only justification for looking at parents of retarded children is that they are taught their responsibilities more quickly and more intensely than most of us. They learn from the beginning that our children have a claim on us even though they do not turn out to be what we expected. Normal children, of course, also always turn out to be quite different than we expected, but we are not made so intensely aware of the implications of that fact in those cases.

Parents of retarded or multiple-handicapped children learn from the beginning they must fight for their children. In this regard it is illuminating to listen to Helen Brown's account of a time soon after the birth of her multiple-handicapped daughter, an account that I suspect could be duplicated by countless other parents of retarded children.

> At home we couldn't discuss Karen. Richard seemed brave and strong. Unknown to me, he and my mother visited Karen at the hospital almost every day. But between us, there was only grief-stricken silence. No one wanted to talk about Karen; no one offered comfort and advice. The specialists were aloof and matter-of-fact. My mother and husband were as overcome as I was. My neighbors—most of them pregnant or new mothers themselves—only brought home to me my loss. I turned at last to the doctor who had delivered Karen and who supplied my only comfort.

"Have another baby as soon as possible," he told me.

"But maybe, just maybe, Karen will come home, and she'll need me."

"Please listen to the experts," he said. "Be brave and strong. You're a perfectly healthy young woman, and there's no reason why you can't have a dozen more children. Let this child go."

I couldn't give up my desperate hope that she would turn out to be perfect and well. I couldn't make the idea of another baby seem like a reality. Only Karen was real, even though I hadn't seen her since she was born.

"You would be ruining your life and your marriage if you tried to bring her home," the doctor said. "Right now she needs constant supervision and medication, and if she survives, there's no telling what she'll be like. Put her out of your mind."

"At least let me see her."

"There's nothing you can do for her. You'd only be breaking your heart."

"She must need her mother. Babies need their mothers."

"She doesn't know the difference, believe me. The best thing to do is forget her."

Wouldn't it have been wonderful — to be able to forget her? If I could have done that, it might have been best, but I was haunted by the memory of her, the child of my dreams, the only two times I had ever seen her: first perfect and beautiful, then red and convulsed, through the window of the hospital nursery.

I tried to forget, but I couldn't.[4]

That such a conversation is not unusual is well-documented in Rosalyn Darling's *Families Against Society*.[5] Darling began her study to test whether in fact handicapped children have the low self-esteem that most theories of self-esteem seem to suggest they should. She soon discovered that their self-esteem was not significantly different from that of normal control groups. On investigating why this might be the case she discovered that if parents of handicapped children regard them positively, then their children are likely to have high self-esteem, regardless of the views of anyone else.

That parents of retarded children learn to regard their children with respect, however, is no simple process. Indeed, Darling found that prior to the birth or later discovery of their child's handicap most parents share our society's general negative judgment about such children. As one of Darling's respondents says, "I knew nothing about mental retardation — just the vague stories one hears when growing up. These were 'people to be shunned.' I was ignorant of any factual knowledge" (Darling 1979, p. 124). It is only through intense day-to-day interaction with their children that parents find the means to challenge and change their own stereotypes of what it means to be handicapped as well as find the means to challenge the stereotypes of our society. Darling's book, therefore, is primarily an account of how parents were taught by their handicapped children to be parents.

Most parents of handicapped children, according to Darling, go through a series of stages which she characterizes from anomie to activism.[6] At first, parents are simply shocked into a state of helplessness by the knowledge that something is seriously wrong with their child. Their feeling of helplessness is only exaggerated by professionals who do not tell them what is wrong with their child in the interest of protecting them from the truth. Not only is the anxiety of parents increased by the evasiveness of many of the professionals, but many parents feel that doctors tend to be overly negative about the description of their child's condition. Thus, Darling quotes some parents reporting: "The doctor called me and said that there was a question about the baby's health, that there was concern over whether we had a 'good baby,' and some doctors seem to think he's mongoloid," and even, "The pediatrician said, 'Your baby has 3M Syndrome. Here's some information you can read about it, but don't worry, she probably won't live' " (Darling 1979, p. 133).

Darling characterizes this first stage as anomie to denote the parents' feelings of helplessness and lack of support in the face of what appears at the time to be an overwhelming tragedy. The temptation of self-pity and a concern for the future quickly become all-consuming for many parents. But interestingly enough this period often tends to be short-lived if the parents receive support from the family and friends and, in particular, if they have interaction with the child. For example, Darling was told:

> I talked to a nurse and then I felt less resentment. I said I was afraid, and she helped me feed the baby. . . . Then my girlfriend came to see me. She had just lost her husband, and we sort of supported each other. . . . By the time she came home, I loved her. When I held her the first time, I felt love and worried if she would live.

As time goes on, you fall in love. You think, "This kid's mine and nobody's gonna take her away from me." I think by the time she was two weeks old I wasn't appalled by her anymore. (Darling 1979, p. 136)

After recovering from their initial anomie, Darling suggests parents begin what she calls a "seekership" phase. The greatest need they feel is for information, not just about their child's condition, but about what can be done. Too often friends and relatives at this point try to help by denying the seriousness of the child's condition. Even more troubling is the common complaint of parents that the medical treatment their children received is not only often inadequate but also dehumanizing. Almost all parents of retarded children report that:

My pediatrician kept after me to put him away [in an institution]. (We finally changed pediatricians.) Our new pediatrician gushed all over us at first. . . . But then, he never touched Billy. I always had to move him for him. We were never left in the waiting room. It was like I was an embarrassment. When Billy was in the hospital, our old pediatrician stuck his head in the door and said, "it's too bad he couldn't go [die]. . . . " The doctors on rounds would talk outside our door and they ripped apart parents who keep their [severely handicapped] children. (Darling 1979, p. 151)

Another parent reported that taking your child to the doctor is like "when you take your dog to the vet . . . not many doctors pick him up and try to communicate with him as a child" (Darling 1979, p. 151).

If Darling's research is anything close to accurate, there does seem to exist a wide discrepancy between the attitudes of pediatricians and parents of handicapped children. Thus, in her interviews with pediatricians, they almost all testified to their dislike of caring for handicapped (and in particular, retarded) children. They usually recommend institutionalization. In the words of one physician, "I have yet to see a mother who has not been adversely affected by having a mongoloid child in the house. Despite the fact that women protest and act in a good, competent way, I really feel that it's affected their lives in a way that robs their being a better person. If one is to think that the object is to make a better life, it interferes with that object. Seeing these people over the years . . . the look in their eyes, their demeanor — it's compensatory, not fulfilling" (Darling 1979, p. 216).

Most parents soon learn not to look for miracles or cures. All they want is to find a competent pediatrician or specialist who will treat their child "like a person." Unfortunately, parents are often forced to spend a great deal of their time simply trying to find a physician who is able to view their child in this manner.

During this period, parents increasingly discover that they do not have great difficulty in learning to accept their children as they learn that they are able to meet their needs. Interestingly enough, this adds to the parents' self-esteem as they realize that they are capable of more than they expected. The difficulty comes not in accepting their own children, but in our society's unwillingness to accept these children as part of our public lives. Parents soon discover that their own matter-of-fact acceptance of their children and their handicaps is not widely shared in our society. They often must learn to deal with the pained embarrassment, if not outright hostility, that results from bringing their children out in public.

Parents learn, however, that public rejection of their children is one of the small obstacles they must encounter. As their children grow older and as their parents seek education, physical, and recreational services, they discover that such services are inadequate or do not exist at all. As one mother put it, they soon realize that "Our society is not geared for the retarded. We used to send them all away and now we don't know what to do with them" (Darling 1979, p. 178). As a result, parents learn it is not enough to try to find the service available for their children. They must learn to fight to establish and create the kind of care their children rightly deserve. Some, Darling denotes, attribute this kind of advocacy for their children to guilt, but she suggests that such "parental behavior is easily understandable within the context of parents trying to 'do their job' as parents in an inhospitable society" (Darling 1979, p. 181).

Thus, parents enter what Darling calls an "advocacy" period as they find they must create institutions and programs to provide better care for their children. They become crusaders willing to challenge the at best sentimental attitude and care offered by our society by demanding their children be treated with respect. It is of interest to note that Darling discovered that often lower-income and less-educated parents become the most effective advocates for their children, as they seem to have had more experience in dealing with unresponsive bureaucracies.

The great strength of parents of retarded children is their lack
of illusion about their children. They refuse to let their children be
destroyed by sentimental kindness that ends only by reinforcing our
stereotypes about what the "retarded are able to do." They demand
that our society provide the training that will allow their children to
attain the level of activity of which they are capable, even if such training
proves painful for their children.

In this respect, the parents of retarded children have often faced
the reality of their situation with more insight than most of us assume
is the case. For example, all of Darling's respondents suggested they
would have preferred that their child not be born with handicaps
because they would not wish their child so burdened. Once their children were born, however, they discovered they loved them no less for
their handicap and gained new confidence in themselves as they learned
to deal with the demands such children placed on them. This confidence, moreover, gave them the strength to take on a much larger
struggle against the ways in which our society ignores or flatly rejects
the retarded.

The extent of that struggle has recently been depicted by John
Gliedman and William Roth in their book *The Unexpected Minority:
Handicapped Children in America*. They point out that the most
decisive disadvantage the handicapped face in our society is not the
most overt forms of discrimination that come through our educational
and economic structures, which are certainly real enough, but the very
categories through which we understand the handicapped. In contrast
to most analyses of the handicapped which suggest that the problem
is providing better medical and social help for the handicapped, Gliedman and Roth argue that the handicapped should be understood as
an oppressed minority group.

It is not that Gliedman and Roth are opposed to the handicapped
getting better medical and educational help, but what is crucial is the
presupposition on which that help is determined. For example, they
suggest that they began their study believing "that the traditional definition of the handicapped child's needs was perfectly satisfactory—that
all that was really required was more of the same kind of services for
handicapped children. Only gradually did we come to see our initial
error. By failing to think through the implications of the 'civil rights
lens' for the child, we had unwittingly committed ourselves to making the same kinds of mistakes about disability that were made about
other groups of disadvantaged children a generation ago."[7]

This mistake, according to Gliedman and Roth, consists in the failure to recognize or understand the implications that a "handicap" is fundamentally a social construction. As a society we tend to diagnose handicaps as diseaselike states. However, this entails a vicious circle.

> Our misconceptions about the incapacitating consequences of a disability cause us to see the person as a deviant, as one who cannot fit into any of the roles assumed by normals in everyday life. Then the culturally determined associations of deviance with disease states encourage us to single out those aspects of the individual that are disease like. By assigning a medical cause to the paraplegic's deviance — his putative inability to assume any normal role in society — lay society denies its responsibility for excluding the individual from normal life.[8]

What we must come to understand, they argue, is that our apparent "objective" perceptions of handicaps as socially incapacitating biological conditions are perceptual products of a prior, and often unconscious, social construction.[9]

Gliedman and Roth note that on the surface this way of identifying the handicapped seems just and fair. After all, to be handicapped is not viewed as punishment (at least not overtly), nor is it invested with mysterious supernatural associations. Rather, we assume that we are taking a scientific approach — that since the handicapped are portrayed as the victims of impersonal accidents, disease processes, and genetic imperfections, stigma and prejudice are out of place. The handicapped are excused because they cannot help being handicapped any more than someone can help being sick. Therefore, what is called for is understanding and assistance.[10]

What we fail to see, however, is that by interpreting handicaps in terms of the medical model, we have in effect robbed the handicapped of what they need most. The medical model obscures the essential fact about the handicapped person's situation, namely, that the disadvantages that result from most handicaps derive more from our society's prejudices than from the handicap itself. The medical model is particularly destructive for the handicapped in that it puts them in a disastrous psychological and sociological situation: they must define themselves as permanently dependent if they are to receive the advantages of the sick role. Moreover, this robs handicapped persons of their most effective means of doing something about their situation, namely, politics. Because issues of health and disease are matters which are thought dealt with primarily in terms of charity, the handicapped are denied the very resource necessary to understand or deal with the discrimination they experience for what it is, namely, they have been robbed unjustly of power that is rightfully theirs and which can only be regained politically. The burden of Gliedman and Roth's presentation is to show that once this has happened, the various professions designed to help the handicapped, often with the best will and enthusiam for the task, are but another form of discrimination as they depoliticize the handicapped person's situation.

Without denying the social nature of any understanding of a "handicap," Gliedman and Roth's point can be misleading if the implication is drawn that all identification of handicaps are arbitrary and discriminating. There is something wrong with someone who is retarded, just as there is something wrong with the fact I have flat feet. The retarded have real disabilities and they need aid, and of the best kind, to help them deal with their handicap.

Gliedman and Roth, however, are right that retardation is a social construction in terms of how a handicap is understood and how it is interpreted to limit the retarded's activity. Moreover, they are right to suggest that retardation, as a social construction, is particularly destructive for anyone so described as it is assumed to describe a condition that determines a person's every activity. Everything we are and do is done as one who is "retarded." What is needed is discriminating forms of judgment that denote those aspects of life and activities where the category of retardation simply is irrelevant. But that, it seems, is exactly what we do not have, and as a result Gliedman and Roth are right to suggest that retardation too often becomes a self-fulfilling prophecy that unfortunately is perpetuated by the very theories and people who want to "help" the retarded.

Parents and the Professional

As I suggested earlier, Gliedman and Roth think that the only source capable of breaking this vicious cycle is for parents of retarded children to reclaim their right to determine the kind of care their children should receive. It is parents, who often have not been schooled on theories about what their retarded children can and cannot do, who are able to demand more from those who would too easily acquiesce to the limitations of the medical model. No one can be around parents of retarded children long, people who, to be sure, have often sought and dealt with one professional after another in the hopes of finding help for their child, without realizing that these are among the few people in our society who have learned to deal with the tyranny of the "expert."

That they have done so is largely because they have learned to trust their own judgment when dealing with their child. To be sure, they are more knowledgeable than most of us and they have learned, often painfully, that experts disagree. However, their fundamental ability to resist the professional comes from their passionate commitment to make the expert see their children as they have learned to see their children, i.e., as fellow members of the human community whose struggle with the limits and possibilities of their existence deserves our most profound respect and support.

I think it would be a mistake, however, to interpret the relationship between the retarded and their parents as only a one-way street. For I have observed that the retarded have often done marvelous things for their parents, not the least of which is their requiring their parents, in their role as advocates, to come in contact with others who are as different from them as their own children. In the process, unlike most of us, their parents have also learned basic political skills for the formation of communities as they learn to work and plan together in order to secure their children a better life.

Even more important to my mind is how parents of retarded children discover what the world is like through their children. The necessity of caring for such children requires us quickly to break through the myths and deceptions that our social order encourages us to accept — one of which is that life is about being a perpetual member of the Pepsi® generation. Our society encourages us to think that we can be a good people without suffering, that we can pursue our own interests with little thought of what it does to others. Parents of children born retarded know better. And because they know better they are able to insist that our society see their children not as permanently ill, but simply as different.

Much more could be said about such matters, but enough has been said to make my basic point, namely, that through their children parents of retarded children are trained to be parents in a manner that illuminates what it means morally to be a parent for anyone. Nothing I have said, of course, commits me to the thesis that parents of the retarded, any more than the retarded themselves, are free from perverse distortions of their role. Indeed, many people unable to face their retarded children abandon them literally or at least psychologically. Or there are parents who unduly emphasize and reinforce their child's handicap as a means to enhance their own status. We all to some extent thrive on the need to be needed and it is hard indeed to learn to force independence on those who seem so dependent.

No doubt other equally subtle and more destructive behavior could be depicted involving the way some parents of retarded children manage themselves and their children. That perversions occur does not show that our commitment to the family as the primary locus for care of children is wrong. Rather, the perversions are but indications of the extraordinary demands that such commitments entail. By calling attention to the way parents of retarded children are taught to be parents, I have tried to remind us how certain kinds of responsibilities give substance to our assumption that the family should have primary responsibility for the rearing of and caring for children.

Before I try to make something out of all this, however, let me qualify an impression that I may have created. For the "heavy" in the above account appears to be the professional—the doctor, researcher, social worker, teacher, and many others. To be sure, many professionals surely deserve the criticism as made, but many do not. Many are dedicated people who see retarded people clearly and often more clearly than parents themselves. Indeed, all parents need help from others, whether they be "professionals" or not, to jar them out of too easily accepted assumptions about the limits or possibilities of their children's capabilities.

The problem with making the professional the bad guy, however, involves a more fundamental mistake than simply slandering many of the dedicated and competent professions who deal with the retarded. For when the professional is made the primary object of criticism, we fail to diagnose adequately our situation. The problem and the dilemma is more profound than simply challenging the dominance of the professional. For the truth is that the state and the professional, who often acts as the agent of the state, have increasingly been called on to be more directly involved in the care of the retarded because the family has simply abdicated its role. But, as I will try to show, that families have done so is not simply because they are morally deficient, though some may be, but because as a society we lack a consensus that can inform expectations as to child care and what kind of support is appropriate for our society and state to provide.

The Dilemma of Care

Therefore, rather than continuing my paean to parents of the retarded, we need to step back and ask some critical questions about what I have been doing. For, in effect, I have used a persuasive example to do the work of argument and in the process belied the ambiguity of our commitment to care for the retarded by and through the family. I have tried to suggest why we rightly think that the family is and should be the primary locus of care for the retarded by calling attention to how the retarded train their parents to care for them. By appealing to the everyday, but in many ways quite heroic, struggle of parents to secure adequate care for their handicapped children, I have reinforced our assumption that the family should have priority for the care of the retarded.

By proceeding by way of example, however, I have weighed the case in a manner that fails to take adequate account of the dilemma raised by focusing on care of the retarded through the family. Simply put, all I have shown is that our society supports the formal commitment that children should be cared for by their parents, but that society does not and cannot require parents to give the kind of care that my examples suggest and which most of us find so admirable. In other words, I have reinforced our assumption that the retarded should be cared for through the agency of the family by suggesting, without adequate support, that such care will be of the kind my examples display.

I can make this more concrete in terms of some of the agonizing dilemmas that occur in almost any hospital with a neonatal unit. Often children are born who, in addition to being retarded, also have some other accompanying difficulty that requires surgical correction if the child is to live. The most famous case is that of a Down's syndrome child born with duodenal atresia whose parents refused the surgery necessary to stop the child from starving to death.

More difficult cases involve questions about how much should be done or how much parents should do to keep alive children suffering from spina bifida. Many assume the parents of the Down's syndrome child were clearly wrong not to secure adequate medical attention for their child, but when confronted by the multiple and severe problems often associated with spina bifada, the case is not so clear and the correct paths not so sure. I am not interested at this point in arguing the case one way or the other; rather, I simply want to point out that if we grant that the family is the primary locus for care of the retarded, this by no means insures that the retarded will receive the kind of care we think they should receive.[11]

A still more troubling issue is raised by programs to prevent retardation. No one would wish that a child be born retarded when it can be avoided through proper prenatal care and adequate infant and early childhood maintenance. But the language of prevention when applied to retardation is more ambiguous than is often recognized.

The problem of prevention can be graphically illustrated by asking whether we, as a society, ought to encourage all women thirty-five and older to undergo amniocentesis. By asking this question, I do not mean to weight the question of abortion one way or the other. Rather, I am simply trying to explore what such a suggestion would mean for our attitudes about the retarded and in particular the responsibilities of parents for them.

For example, it is quickly becoming a general assumption that a woman thirty-five or older should have amniocentesis. As a result, anyone who has a retarded child in later life is viewed with a good deal of suspicion, if not outright hostility. After all, they should have known better and taken the appropriate steps. But why do we think that? Why do we assume that it is the task of parents to avoid having children who may be retarded? Or perhaps better, how far do we think that people ought to go in order to avoid having retarded children?

Moreover, our concern with prevention of the retarded may have unanticipated social policy implications. It has been our assumption that a reduction in the number of retarded children will translate into more public dollars for their care. However, this by no means follows, as the diminishing social budget we face over the next few years might well turn in the other direction. The fewer who need to be cared for might mean that our society would find it less costly simply to make parents do the best they can, and if they abdicate this responsibility, the state can warehouse these children more easily. Or still more troubling, as amniocentesis becomes more common, some may think they have little responsibility to support with public money a mistake the parents could have easily avoided.

Perhaps even more troubling are the moral implications of amniocentesis as a public policy. For public policy involves not just issues of distribution but also assumptions about what kind of people we ought to be. Does amniocentesis imply that we should be willing to be parents only if we can assume we are working with a "perfect" child? And if so, how are we to determine what such a child should look like?

By raising these issues I do not mean to suggest that amniocentesis should never be used, but I raise these questions about amniocentesis and the other issues only to illustrate my contention that our appeal to the family as the locus for the care of the retarded simply is not sufficient to tell us how the family should care for the retarded. Indeed, as I have tried to suggest, the commitment to the family in itself can as easily result in individual retarded children receiving less than adequate care and may mean that the retarded receive even less support as the object of social policy.

Thus we find ourselves in a dilemma. We are inheritors of a tradition that presumes that the family is our central social institution for the care of children, but we have no idea what the family should be. This dilemma, however, serves to remind us that the family is not an end in itself or an isolatable social entity, but requires moral direction and support from a community. The family does not exist just to exist, but like any other significant institution it needs purposes and tasks. This is exactly what our society is unsure about, since to specify tasks for the family with any kind of moral specificity appears as a threat to our "freedom." As a result, we talk much and loudly about the value of the family in our society, having little idea why it in fact has worth.

In this respect, issues raised by the relation of the family and the retarded are but one aspect of the larger problem of the status of the family in our society. We are often told the family is in crisis, but there is little consensus about the nature of cause of the crisis. Indeed, many deny that there is any crisis at all, calling attention to the fact that the family remains very strong, although it is presently experiencing transition and change from past configurations. It is not my intention to enter this debate, but only to suggest that if there is a crisis, it is fundamentally a moral one. Our most basic problem is that we are no longer sure what we are doing when we have children or how we should raise them.

It is an irony that there is no better example of this than Kenneth Keniston's *All Our Children*, a book prepared by the Carnegie

Council on the Family with the express interest of ensuring the continued strength of the family in our society.[12] Keniston and his colleagues conclude that the family simply cannot be, if it ever was, a self-sufficient unit, and thus argue that all families today need help in raising their children.[13] The kind of lives parents are leading, and the lives they are preparing their children to live, are so demanding and complex that parents cannot have — and indeed should not have — traditional kinds of direct supervision of their children.

This does not mean, according to Keniston, that parents have no role in the raising of their children. Rather, they have a demanding new role: theirs is now the task of choosing, meeting, talking with, and coordinating the experts, the technology, and the institutions which help bring up their children. The specific work involved is familiar to any parent: consultations with teachers, finding good health care, trying to monitor television watching, and so on. "No longer able to do it all themselves, parents today are in some ways like the executives in a large firm — responsible for the smooth coordination of the many people and processes that must work together to produce the final product."[14]

I have no interest in trying to deny the descriptive power of Keniston's new understanding of parental responsibility, but at the same time what strikes one is the moral vacuousness of this vision of the family.[15] The idea of the parent as an executive hardly does justice to the kind of commitment we saw exemplified by the parents of retarded children. Indeed, exactly what makes those parents so impressive is their willingness to challenge our society and the "experts" on grounds that they, as parents, know better that their children should not be abandoned by subjecting them to the limits of our technology.

Interestingly, Gliedman and Roth's study of discrimination against handicapped children in our society was part of the same Carnegie study as Keniston's. It would seem that the underwriting of the rearing of children by professionals recommended by Keniston would be exactly the kind of strategy that Gliedman and Roth find so disastrous for handicapped children. They are clearly aware of this but try to maintain a consistency with Keniston's metaphor of parents as executives by suggesting that parents "must have power — the kind of power that comes with occupying a position of administrative authority in a large organization. Without it, even the best-intentioned attempts to reform the way professionals deliver their services risk frustration. For most people — all but the most wealthy, clever, and influential — this power must spring from the same source as that of the administrator — the group. Perhaps more than anything else, it is essential that parents of handicapped children organize themselves into self-help groups."[16]

While I am certainly not against "self-help groups," I think that such a suggestion is hardly sufficient to balance what is in effect the moral abdication of parents warranted by Keniston's recommendation. Indeed at a more profound level, I think there is a great difficulty with Gliedman and Roth's attempt to frame the issue of the discrimination against handicapped children as a civil rights issue. For to put the issue that way makes it appear that "handicapped children" are an "oppressed minority" who are independent of their parents. Yet this is exactly what they are not. In fairness to Gliedman and Roth, however, one can easily understand their resort to a civil rights appeal in as much as there appears to be no other moral categories that would suggest why our society should underwrite the attempt of parents to secure adequate care for their retarded children.

But the very moral presuppositions, i.e., assumptions about rights and equality, implied by the language of civil rights fails to give expression to the profound moral commitments involved in parents' struggles to care for their retarded children. For example, we often assume that to be treated equally is to be treated justly, but on reflection we discover that is not the case. For often the language of equality, especially in our society, only works by reducing us to a common denominator, which can be repressive or disrespectful. This can be seen clearly in terms of blacks' struggle for civil rights. This struggle began with a justified call to be treated equally, to have the opportunity to enjoy the same rights of all Americans that blacks were denied on the basis of color. But black Americans soon discovered that it was not enough to be treated equally if that treatment meant they must forget what it means to be black. For who they are as blacks represents a history that should be cherished and enhanced. No one wants to pay the price of being treated equally if that means they must reject who they are — that is, if they must lose their roots in the process of becoming "free" or "equal."

The commitment of parents to their retarded children in this respect involves a more profound and richer sense of community than the language of equality can provide. For the retarded call us toward a community of diversity and difference where that difference is not used as the basis of arbitrary discrimination. In this sense, the retarded are a concrete test of the moral implications of a society's willingness to let the differences occasioned by our familial heritages flourish. A society that takes seriously the commitment to the family as the civilizing agency for the rearing of children is one that has learned that equality must not occasion policies that force us to forget or hide our differences — indeed, even the differences that result from being retarded — help each of us to flourish.

But there should be no mistake about it: such a community and society that thrives on differences is a hard enterprise to sustain. We are creatures who fear differences. The fact that the other is not as we are is more often perceived as a threat than as a gift. The only solution is to make others as much like ourselves as possible, or to make them live apart from us, or if necessary, not to live at all. Thus, whites fear blacks, men fear women, and all of us fear the retarded.

Only when we realize this have we reached the point where we can understand the depth of the dilemma raised by our commitment to care for the retarded by and through their parents. Our problem is that we have no philosophy of public morality through which we are able to articulate the kind of commitment we find witnessed in the lives of parents who have learned through their children to be parents. I do not think there is any easy solution to this problem. Rather, I think what we must do is let the witness of such parents guide our way, as they stand as a beacon to remind us what it means to be a parent no matter what our child may be like.

But that they are witnesses only indicates the tenuousness of our situation. How long can we expect to be graced with such presence when we even lack the moral language to express the commitments their lives display? Perhaps, however, in the interim the best thing we can do is to make public these remarkable, but no less ordinary, families.[17]

NOTES

1. John Gliedman and William Roth, *The Unexpected Minority: Handicapped Children in America* (New York, 1979), p. 104. My paginations are from the page proof copy of this book.

2. Of course this needs to be qualified to some extent as we do not

assume that parents can do anything to their children they wish — thus we prevent parents from gross physical abuse.

3. For a more extended analysis of this claim see my *A Community of Character: Toward a Constructive Christian Social Ethic* (Notre Dame, Ind.: University of Notre Dame Press, 1981).

4. Helene Brown, *Yesterday's Child* (New York: Signet Books, 1976), pp. 33–34.

5. Rosalyn Darling, *Families Against Society* (Beverly Hills, Ca.: Sage Library of Social Research, 1979). All page references will appear in text. For an even more powerful testimony by parents about their struggles to have their retarded children regarded and treated with respect see *Parents Speak Out: Then and Now*, edited by H. R. Turnbull and Ann Turnbull (Columbus, Ohio: Charles Merrill, 1985). The constant theme of the Turnbull's remarkable book is how parents had to fight with professionals to see their children as they had learned to see them.

6. Darling's work has the disadvantage of being shaped by the rather tiresome and distracting methodological concerns — not the least of which is the language of stages. I have no doubt, as anyone can testify who has been around parents of retarded children or who has read some of the excellent accounts by parents of the struggle with their children, that many do go through the kind of stages Darling suggests. But this is a highly relative matter that is not easily reduced to language of stages. In many ways it might have been better for me simply to have used the more biographical accounts such as Greenfeld or White, but Darling's book has the advantage of reporting the responses of a large group of parents. I, therefore, decided to use her book, as the parents Darling quotes often say more than her methodological structure is able to bring out.

7. Gliedman and Roth, *The Unexpected Minority*, p. x.

8. Ibid., p. 11.

9. Ibid., p. 15. The notion of "social construction" is highly problematic when used as a general account of all knowledge, but I think Gliedman and Roth use the notion in an appropriately modest way.

10. Ibid., p. 20.

11. For a more extended discussion of these issues, however, see my *Truthfulness and Tragedy* (Notre Dame, Ind.: University of Notre Dame Press, 1977), pp. 147-183; and my "Selection of Children to Live or Die: An Ethical Analysis of the Debate between Dr. Lorber and Dr. Freeman on the Treatment of Meningomyelocele," in *Death, Dying, and Euthanasia*, ed. Dennis Horan and David Mall (Washington, D.C.: University Press of America, 1977), pp. 228–249.

12. Kenneth Keniston, *All Our Children: The American Family under Pressure* (New York: Harcourt Brace Jovanovich, 1977).

13. Ibid., p. 22.

14. Ibid., p. 17.

15. For analysis as well as critique of this view of the family, see Christopher Lasch, *Haven in a Heartless World* (New York: Basic Books, 1977). Lasch points out that much of the social theory and accompanying social service professions created to help the family in fact were anti-family insofar as they reinforced the idea that the family's primary function was to be an emotional haven of privacy in a forbidding society. The more the family corresponded to that image the more it needed "experts" to prop it up, since we increasingly lost the skills of familial survival.

16. Gliedman and Roth, *The Unexpected Minority*, pp. 123–124.

17. I would like to thank Anne Hauerwas and Mark Sherwindt for their criticism of an earlier version of this paper.

12

Community and Diversity: The Tyranny of Normality

It is great honor for me to be given the opportunity to speak at such an occasion. For I have no claim or right to be heard by you. Those of you who have retarded children and/or work with retarded children already know far more than anything I could say. Moreover, you have felt the sadness, suffering, and joy of being, having, and working with retarded citizens that I have not. It is an honor that you have asked me to speak to you, since I feel that day in and day out you speak much more eloquently to me.

Therefore, I must speak to you as an "outsider" who has had the privilege of being with those on the inside. Usually there is not much advantage to being an "outsider," but at least it gives me the opportunity to see what you are doing through fresh eyes. For I have noticed that those that have retarded children and work with the retarded are often so busy doing, they have little time to reflect on why, how, or what they are doing. This is, of course, not an unusual thing to have happen. It has been remarked that if fish ever developed intelligence and began to codify and describe their environment, one of the last things they would notice would be the water. Therefore, as an outsider, I want to try to say a few things tonight that may help you notice what kind of water you folks are swimming in, in terms of that which binds us together—namely, our commitment to the support of those born not like us that we describe with the unhappy word "retarded."

Now I am bold enough to take this tack because I think that one of our difficulties is that you do not know how to describe why it is that we share this commitment. In other words, I think that our culture

This talk was delivered at the 1977 annual dinner of the Council for the Retarded of St. Joseph County, Indiana.

too often offers us no account, or worse a misleading account, of this commitment. Each of you has developed your special, or perhaps better, your personal account of why this commitment is so significant. Such accounts often are as profoundly simple as what it means to be a parent, or they may involve convictions about one's own vocation. But as important as our personal accounts are, we need more if the existence and care of the retarded are to be seen as important for the outsiders. We need an account that helps give, not only those involved with the retarded, but also those who only support that involvement indirectly, a sense that this is a good and essential task for everyone in our community.

Moreover, when we lack such accounts or stories about what we are doing, we often are captured by destructive accounts. On the personal level, for example, we can tell ourselves false stories about being sacrificial parents—to the detriment of our children. We know this is dangerous because we learn how hard it is to make a sacrifice without making those we sacrificed for pay for our effort. Or we can be captured by destructive accounts about the retarded—namely, they are more innocent or sweet than other children or people. That is a terrible story to have to live out, because who wants to go through life being innocent and sweet.

At the social level we also can run into some misleading claims about what we are doing. For example, many of us fighting for better treatment for the retarded use the language of securing the rights of the retarded. To be sure, the language of rights has a moral and social significance, but we must use it carefully, for too often in our political system it is the battle cry of one interest group against another. When used in this manner it transforms what should be our society's moral commitment into an issue comparable to a conflict between business and labor. If we are to use the language of rights, we must be clear that we do so only as a means to protect the retarded from those who would treat them, for either cruel or sentimental reasons, with less than respect.

I think it is important, therefore, that we remember that the language of rights is dependent on a more profound sense of community that forms our commitment to the retarded. Speaking as the "outsider," I want to suggest that the retarded help us understand some crucial things about what it means to be a community that enhances us all. Put differently, many talks about the retarded are about what we should be doing for them, but I am suggesting that they do something for us that we have hardly noticed. Namely, they force us to recognize that we are involved in a community life that is richer than our official explanations and theories give us the skill to say.

For example, we usually associate movements toward justice in our society with the language of equality. We assume to be treated equally is to be treated justly, but on reflection we may discover that is not the case. Often the language of equality only works by reducing us to a common denominator that can be repressive or disrespectful. This can perhaps be seen most clearly in terms of the black struggle for civil rights. Namely, that struggle began with a justified call to be treated equally — to have the opportunity to enjoy the same rights of all Americans that blacks were denied on basis of their color. But black Americans soon discovered that it was not enough to be treated equally if that treatment meant they must forget what it means to be black. Being black is just who they are. To be "black" is to be part of a history that should be cherished and enhanced. No one wants to pay the price of being treated equally if that means they must reject who they are — that is, if they must reject their roots. We find the same kind of movement today among those born Hungarian, Polish, Spanish, or (the ultimate good) Texan. In other words, none of us want to be treated equally if that means we lose our distinctiveness.

Now it seems to me that our commitment to having the retarded in our society embodies a richer sense of community than the language of equality provides. For the retarded, in a profounder way than being black, Hungarian, Pole, or even Texan, call us toward a community of diversity and difference. Such a community is a community of equality, but not in the way that equality makes us forget our differences. Rather in community of equality our differences help each of us to flourish exactly as different people.

There should be no mistake about it, a community of diversity that enhances differences is indeed a hard enterprise to sustain. We are creatures that fear difference. The fact that the other is not as we are means that there may be something wrong with us. The only solution is to make them as much like us as possible or to make them live apart.

Most of us learn to deal with this demand to be like everyone else — we have the power. It should be said, however, that we are not nearly as successful as we think, as too often we voluntarily accept the other's definition of us. The most stringent power we have over another is not physical coercion but the ability to have the other accept our definition of them. But the retarded are often in the unfortunate position of not having the power to resist those who would make them like us.

This consideration, I think, must make us a little cautious about being too enthusiastic about the "principle of normalization" that is currently so popular among those who work with the retarded. It is of course true that the retarded deserve to do what they are able — to dress themselves, to spend their own money, to decide to spend their money foolishly or wisely, to date, to fall in love, and so on. But the demand to be normal can be tyrannical unless we understand that the normal condition of our being together is that we are all different. If we are to be a good community we must be one that has convictions substantive enough not to fear our differences and, indeed, to see that we would not be whole without the other being different than us.

Besides the gift of difference and its importance for community, it seems to me that the retarded also help us to see how to be different without regret. It is one of the conditions of modern consciousness that we all feel that we have suffered injustice or that we are ruled by powers not of our own making. Put graphically, we all tend to think of ourselves, at least in some moods, as victims.

Now I suspect that we have all in one way or another suffered injustice, but there is a problem with thinking of ourself as a victim. Because once we take on that role it may make us misdescribe what our problem is and we look for help in the wrong place. It makes us acquiesce too readily to our condition, assuming that there is nothing we can do until something is done out there.

On anyone's scale of those who have suffered some of the worst injustices across human societies, surely the retarded would be close to the top. But by what must almost be considered special grace, they do not think of themselves as victims. And I do not think that this is simply because they fail to understand what has happened to them. Rather it seems to me that they understand that we all get "stuck with" certain limits and certain societies. I am "stuck with" being a Texan and being bald, but the question is what I am going to do with being so "stuck." To be sure, some social conditions make some things we are "stuck with" unjust, and we ought not to tolerate that. But finally we must all learn, as it seems to me that the retarded often do better than any of us, that ultimately we are all "stuck with" ourselves, and that is not a bad thing.

For the limits we are "stuck with" are as much a source of our difference as are our talents. We are valuable to one another, not in spite of our talents, but because of them. Even though the retarded represent a limit in our communities, they also represent a limit we cannot be without. For without them and the attitude they bring to their limits, we would all be the poorer.

For example, let me suggest what I have observed the retarded have done for their parents. First, they have required their parents to join together and come in contact with others who are as different from them as their own children. In the process they discover they have interests beyond simply sharing similar children. They share similar pains and sufferings, joy and triumphs that join them in community more profound than a mere association. That is the reason they can risk disagreement, because they know they are bound together in profound and lasting ways.

Secondly, parents of retarded children discover what the world is like through their children. Their children provide them with the means to break through the myths and illusions that our social order wants us to accept — namely, that life is about being members of the Pepsi® generation. Or society encourages us to think that one can be a good people without suffering, that we can pursue our own interests with little thought of what it does to others. But parents of children born retarded know better. No people in society can be good without paying a price. The crucial thing is how we help and support one another as we are each called upon to pay that price.

Or on a more mundane, but no less important level, I have noticed the parents of retarded children know a lot more about politics than most of us. You know who your state congress person is and you know how to get in touch with her or him. You know the institutions that sustain and run us and you learn how to make them work for the good. Without your children you would be just as uninformed as the average American about the social system that forms our lives.

Finally, one of the things your children have done for you is to help you be free from the tyranny of the professional. Now this involves arduous training and struggle that is never over, but generally you do better at it than most of us. For example, almost no one in our society has the guts to ask doctors for a second opinion, but you do. You have learned to do that because you have learned that professionals can be wrong and you are not going to let your child suffer because of the ego of a professional.

In fact, what parents of retarded children learn to do is trust their own good judgment, and that is a hard thing to do in a society which assumes that there is an expert about everything. We all need help from one another, but not because some are "experts" and others are not, but because good communities learn to use the experience that comes from different functions. But we must remember that when it comes to our children we are all experts and we should not let a professional determine what our child is, means, or can do.

Now I have been speaking as an outsider, but in closing I think it best to let an insider speak. In a book called *Journey*, Suzanne and Robert Massie describe their struggle to keep alive and raise their hemophilic son. Mrs. Massie, pregnant with her third child, discovers the development and increasing accuracy of prenatal diagnosis. And of course the question arises whether she would have welcomed such counseling before the birth of her hemophilic son. She says,

> Perhaps, even very soon, premarital genetic counseling will be routine. No doubt this will be useful and helpful. But I couldn't help thinking as I heard those discussions among doctors, how glad I was that I had not been counseled BEFORE. For one thing, it is such an uneven relationship—the doctor, wearing a white coat and radiating scientific superiority, advising an untechnical, uninformed, frightened lay person. There is little training for such counseling in medical schools today—doctors are left to their own prejudices. Much of what passes under the guise of medical counseling really consists only of saying no; of advising the safe way, the way of least resistance. Not long ago, I attended a medical symposium and heard a famous geneticist talk learnedly about the need for "objective" counseling in cases of genetic disease. Fine. Then he concluded his remarks with this highly subjective sentence: "I cannot imagine a family who would not WISH TO AVOID the emotional and financial stress imposed upon them when a hemophiliac is born."

> I wonder. Suppose someone had talked to me this way? Suppose I had been told before I was married that I was a carrier for hemophilia and therefore should not have any children? Suppose I had been ad-

vised to adopt children? Personally, I am profoundly grateful that I was not told, that I did not have to make the decision of whether to have or not to have Bobby. Looking back at myself, a newly married young woman, unfamiliar with the feelings of a mother, I think, had I been asked, I would have said no. No one wants to suffer. Everyone is afraid of challenge and sacrifice. This is normal and known. If someone had asked me, "do you want to walk through fire?" the answer would have been no, of course not. I am afraid of being burned. Yet once in the fire, I fought to get through it and it is at least possible to think that the experience left me stronger. It is not the struggle but the unknown that we fear most. If genetic counseling is to be meaningful, then not only must those counseled be informed of the purely scientific facts, they must also be encouraged to believe in themselves, in their own capacities to live and grow. They must be counseled not only to FEAR, but to be brave enough to live with the question.

Without questions, would we ever search for answers? A child with a genetic illness is a perpetual question, pushing us to seek answers to this dilemma of nature and God.

It was with all these vivid impressions that I waited for my third child.

I can add nothing to this, for if an "outsider" is wise, he should know when to shut up and let the "insiders" speak. But what I hope I have at least suggested is that the struggle, the pain, the suffering, and the joy of the "insiders" is not insignificant for those of us on the outside. For without you and your children, our communities would be less rich in the diversity of folk that we need in order to be good communities.

Index